For my parents,
Stanley and Lois Hankins

Contents

Contents

Acknowledgments

I'm grateful. Cancer came and tried to take it all, but each of you came and you gave. And gave. And gave. With faces toward the east, you stood with me as we watched the colors change and waited for the dawning. Thank you to:

Vicki Crumpton, my editor, and all those at Revell. Each of the 1.6 million people diagnosed with cancer last year has a story to share—and you gave a voice to this one.

Sarah J. Freese and Greg Johnson at WordServe Literary Agency. Thank you for believing in this book.

Patrick M. Finn. I entered your college class at the age of forty-eight with a dream to stop waiting for "some day" in regard to writing. You taught me that writing is giving voice to what people cannot say or are afraid to say.

Joan C. Webb, writing and life coach. Your listening heart is like a cup of cold water for a weary soul, giving strength for the next step.

My dad, Stanley Hankins. When I was a child, you corrected my grammar and red-inked my letters home from camp. My editor thanks you. As an adult, you celebrated my decision to join you as a teller of stories. One of my biggest desires is to hold an audience, like you did, with only words.

My mom, Lois Hankins. Besides brown eyes, I hope my children inherit these three things from you: love of family, faith in God, and grace under pressure. Thank you for teaching me to sing songs in the night.

Our church home at Trinity Christian Fellowship. I can't imagine doing this life of faith without you.

Chandler Relay for Life. Cancer has touched us all, yet from each of you I have learned how to celebrate life, to remember, and to fight back.

My friends, friends of my parents, and our extended family—too numerous to name. You lived out the verse, "I was sick and you visited me."[1] Thank you for being the hands and feet of Jesus to my parents, to my family, and to me.

My siblings: Phil, Renae, and Lisa. We shared our parents for more than half a century and now we collectively hold the memories of our time with them. I am thankful every day I am not an only child.

Our children and their spouses: Nate and Rachel, Aleah and Todd, Katelyn, Zachary. One of my strongest beliefs is that people's stories belong to them. You have given permission for our story to be shared. Thank you for trusting me with the words.

Our grandchildren: Micah, Madelyn, and Benjamin. I see you in the distance. I promise I will run like your lives depend on it.

My husband, Kevin. When we spoke vows over thirty-five years ago, we never could have imagined the difficult beauty that would be part of our story. I am so glad God wrote us together into the pages. I love you.

Jesus. I have heard you in desert skies, in the lives of your people, in your written Word, and in purple lavender. Your pursuing love is amazing. For your purposes, the door to this story has been thrown wide open. I am grateful.

Introduction

I thirst for a sliver of shadow.

The desert sun flares white through the window next to the only available table at the coffee shop where I sit waiting for a friend. In the parking lot, each two-year-old sapling has a car parked under it, the three-inch width of shade spreading long across blistering vehicle chassis. After three days of 110-degree heat, shade is a priceless commodity.

I shift my body away from the relentless burn. I glance at my watch.

My friend is late.

I sip my chai latte, wishing I would have strayed from habit and ordered something iced. The hint of cinnamon and cream does nothing to soothe me.

I pull out my phone. No messages. I know my friend will come if she can. She promised to take a morning nap so she would have the strength to meet me.

I see her coming toward the front door and rush to open it.

Keep smiling, I tell myself. *Don't appear shocked. Keep smiling.*

I give my friend a one-arm hug, careful of her gaunt frame. She grabs me close, collarbones and ribs poking. Her breath is warm on my neck. Does she cling to me? Am I the one holding her?

I offer her the seat away from the sunbeam, but she sits directly in the light and pulls a thin sweater tighter around her shoulders.

"I can't get warm," she says.

I nod. How could I forget my own days of treatment, when radiation fried away my inner thermostat and I shivered wherever I went? Long pants and a sweater became my dearest companions in an air-conditioned theater and nothing was as physically painful as the freezer section of the grocery store, where I quickly grabbed vanilla ice cream and orange juice and rushed over several aisles to warm up next to the rotisserie chicken and right-out-of-the-oven French bread.

My friend asks about my children. I have to turn my ear to hear her forced words. Her voice is raspy. Low. The cancer has spread to her lungs.

She is trying so hard not to disappear, yet she is so faintly here.

We chat for several minutes while the barista whips out espressos and lattes, the scent of coffee mingling with our words. We talk about the weather. Our husbands. Summer plans. Mundane life. Beautiful, ordinary life.

She is the one who brings up her health. "I'm done," she tells me.

"With treatment?" I ask.

"Yes."

A chill runs through me. Wasn't it only four months ago when someone else I loved told me those exact words?

"Is your family done?" I ask.

"Not all of them."

"That's tough."

She agrees. "I am not afraid of eternity, just the process of getting there."

I reach for trembling hands. Her thin fingers cling. Tight. I stumble to reassure, to speak of hard truth found in my own desert wanderings. "I don't know if you will get an easy, gentle ending or a hard, painful one," I say, "but this I can promise you—Jesus will be there in either case."

Her fingers squeeze harder, grasp for difficult reality.

"And He will be there for your family," I say, "for your children. It will be hard, but He will not abandon them either."

I gulp down grief. Memories. "I know," I say. Clear my throat. "I know."

She nods. "That's why I wanted to meet with you."

I gaze into eyes too large in a thin face. I wonder at the depth of what I see. Desperation? No, that is not the right word. Her gaze doesn't waver. She doesn't blink.

Surrender?

Yes, I decide. That is what I perceive, and I bow my head at the pain of that realization. I have seen the same determined finality in others who have fought long, hard battles with this insidious disease that comes like a thief to take it all.

I know my friend wants reassurance that it is okay to be done, to surrender—not to cancer but to a God who has loved her before the beginning of time. She seeks support in this uncharted wilderness place from one who is only a few steps ahead in her own sojourning.

I ponder what to tell her. Having cancer redefined life for me. Watching my mom endure pain from her cancer made me rethink my views on strength. Sitting next to my dad as he faced eternity without fear gave me new thoughts about courage. Meeting people wearing head scarves and proudly displaying their scars caused me to reevaluate my view of beauty. Facing eternity with those whose journey was ending challenged my definitions of hope and faith. Being surrounded by family, community, and a loving, pursuing God expanded my thoughts of belonging.

I remember at the beginning of my journey when I thought I needed to do it on my own, even shutting out my own husband—so determined, yet so foolish.

I inch my chair toward the light until I share the sunbeam with my friend. I fix my eyes on her face, for I have learned that sometimes the greatest act of compassion we offer the dying is not to look away.

One

Cancer Makes a House Call

The clouds gather on a ninety-two-degree day while Mom and Dad help me with the yard work. Dad mentions the gray sky, atypical for this time of year. We are several months away from the shifting winds that bring the life-giving monsoon rains later in the summer. My parents are visiting from their country home near Albert Lea, Minnesota. Dad trims the oleander bushes, the soft pink flowers littering the grass at his feet, while Mom and I rake the rock around the citrus trees.

I answer my cell phone on the first ring.

"Are you sure?" I ask. "Yes. I can come in tomorrow."

"Is that the doctor?" Mom asks when I drop the phone to my side. I stare at her. Numb. The morning sun blisters hot, but I tremble.

"It's cancer." I want to say more, to soften the blow from the test results we've been waiting for, but it is all I can get through my tight throat. I bend double, every particle of air knocked from my body. Mom's arms surround me. Dad's hand squeezes my shoulder, as emotion overwhelms me.

One thought comes into focus: *I need to call my husband, Kevin.*

Mom sniffles as I stare at my phone. How am I going to tell him I have the same disease that killed both his parents? Must worst nightmares be repeated? I punch in his number with freeze-frame fingers.

Kevin answers immediately. "Hello?" In the background, I hear him shuffling papers on his desk.

I clear my throat. Nothing comes out. I am weightless, falling down a rabbit hole, but instead of the white rabbit, I see the doctor in scrubs as he inserted the biopsy needle into my right breast. "You're going to feel a slight pinch," the doctor said.

Instead of a pinch, I feel a punch. A punch right in the center of my life.

"Hello?"

I can't speak. All I can do is sob. Cancer has stolen my words.

———

Sleep becomes illusive, as questions drive me from my bed. As the questions multiply, sleep subtracts, and I struggle to comprehend the incomprehensible.

Why? Why me? Why cancer? Why now? With no family history, I never thought I'd get cancer. I obeyed each and every one of the "How Not to Get Cancer Rules": I consumed healthy foods, exercised regularly, never smoked, and ate my canned peas as a child. Surely that should get me points for something if there was any fairness in the world. But I began to wonder about the whole fairness thing in elementary school when I noticed the pretty girls were allowed cuts in the lunch line. Sometimes life stinks, and since I grew up downwind from a pig farm, I know what I am talking about. Having cancer ranks up there with the smelliest of days.

Along with the questions comes a crushing onslaught of too much information. My brain swims with words like *ductal carcinoma, stages, genetic testing, lumpectomy,* and *possible mastectomy.* Doctors and specialists discuss options, but eventually, all I hear is "Yada, yada . . . CANCER . . . Will I die? . . . yada, yada." A Google search on breast cancer results in 214 million posts to choose from—214 million! How can one person process that amount of data?

Informing our married son, Nate, and fourteen-year-old son, Zach, is difficult, but telling our college-aged daughter, Aleah, and sixteen-year-old daughter, Katelyn, is a million times more difficult, knowing they can no longer check "no" on future medical forms asking if there is a history of breast cancer in the family. I grieve in places, as a mother, I never knew existed.

I call my siblings. Close friends. I tell the story again and again. People cry. *Does rewinding and repeating make it more real?* In the few days following my diagnosis, cancer multiplies to touch everyone I love. *Can't we be actors in a different reality series?*

"Don't tell our teachers," the younger two plead, not wanting to be labeled as The Kids Whose Mom Has Cancer. "People will treat us weird." We acquiesce as their eighth- and tenth-grade years near completion, not realizing how much the silence would wear on them.

We stumble through days. Tests. Doctor appointments. In the swirling numbers of blood counts, days until treatment, and life expectancy, numbers escape Katelyn, who no longer finds algebra relevant. Or English. Or studying for finals. Cancer to her means death, having already lost two grandparents to the disease.

Before I can schedule an appointment at her high school to finally bring the teachers into the cancer loop, Katelyn can't contain the secret any longer and unloads the entire story. As does Zach. "Mom has cancer." They inform the English teacher. Science teacher. Friends.

Storm clouds can only hold so long before bursting.

My children find relief in words shared, but I choose a different course. My heart keeps it all tight. Close. I *will* hold the family together. I hang on to strength. My strength. I will kick cancer in the teeth and get on with my life. I am strong. Stupid strong.

I escape to the desert.

The blast of heat hits me full in the face as I open the door of my Toyota Highlander and step out on the gravel road at the Pima Canyon access at South Mountain. Not yet 5:00 a.m., the parking lot is already filling with mountain bikers and hikers trying to catch the cooler morning temperatures.

I kick off my flip-flops and lace up a pair of running shoes. I slip my hydration pack over my shoulders and snap the belt around my waist, adjusting the nozzle so I can easily reach the water during my workout. Mollie, my terrier-retriever pound puppy, waits for me to connect her leash before we head toward the trailhead, our feet kicking up dust on the dirt service road. The bordering brittlebush droops tired and thirsty. Heat wears everything—and everyone—down.

I have been coming to this trail more years than I can remember. I never meant to live in the desert this long. My husband and I, with a newborn son, moved to Chandler, Arizona, from the Boundary Waters Canoe Area in upper Minnesota, a wilderness of endless lakes and easy water. We came for a season.

Three more children and the season became a decade. And another. And another. Sometimes a season becomes a lifetime.

Through the years I wrestled under blistering sun. Complained. Whined. I grimaced when I stepped out of air-conditioned coolness into sweat-dripping sauna heat. I languished in the endless brown and muted green. My soul longed for one drop of color.

On the trail, Mollie's ears perk up and I follow her gaze to a paloverde, the tree's green bark casting a strange lime color in the dawning. A rabbit rests in the shadows, its long ears twitching as he senses the danger in my rust-colored mutt's interest. Its black tail identifies the bunny as a jackrabbit, not a white-tailed cottontail.

I whisper a command and Mollie sits at my feet, her eyes alert. I pull out my pocket-sized camera and crouch low for a better angle. Mollie whimpers and the jack bounds away, doing what a jackrabbit always does—attempting to outrun an enemy. His black tail is the last thing I see before one final long leap takes him over the horizon.

Down the road I see the crumbled ruins of two stone buildings built during the Great Depression. I tug Mollie's leash toward the trailhead off to the right. I glance at my watch. Later in the day I need to meet with my surgeon and set an appointment for surgery. When my feet hit the narrow path, I start to run. My questions chase me as I speed through the desert.

———

"Why have you brought us out of Egypt to die here in the wilderness?"[1] the desert wanderers asked Moses. I wander under a different desert sun, but the same question festers in my mind. *Why have you brought me out to wilderness—the desert—to die?*

The book of Exodus weaves a tale of the Israelites' escape from slavery under the leadership of Moses and their subsequent journey through the desert. Along the way they complained. Whined. Longed to go back to the place from where they had come.

Perhaps desert stories don't change much in the telling.

Four hundred years of slavery had toughened their muscles as they performed the backbreaking work of making bricks for Pharaoh's endless building projects. Four hundred years of slavery had also toughened their hearts.

Unanswered questions have a way of doing that if we are not careful.

After waiting so many years for the answers to their questions, the Israelites made a joint decision to carve their own path. *God has specific instructions for us to obey? Yeah, right. We have a better idea.* Their better idea bought them a forty-year tour of the desert until all who disobeyed were buried in desert sands. But the story did not end there.

God did not abandon them.

"He did not take away the pillar of cloud by day, nor the pillar of fire by night, from before the people."[2] In a confusing land of countless sand dunes, without streetlights or road signs, God provided His own GPS. A pillar of fire by night. For protection. For warmth. For light.

And during the day? A cloud—the largest shade umbrella that ever existed. The shade covered each and every one of them.

Grandmas. Grandpas. The newborn babies and the boys playing hide-and-seek among the dunes. The mothers searching for another manna recipe. The fathers standing on the lookout for enemy marauders. Under the covering, the Israelites knew where to go. They stood protected from the heat and the elements. The desert travelers only had to look up. And follow.

"Why did you bring us out to the desert to die?"

God never answered their questions. At least not with words. God answered their questions with protection. With direction. With presence.

With shade.

What if God does not answer my questions? Is it possible I too can find Him of endless cloud and covering shadow?

Several years ago, at a family reunion on my mom's side, my aunt collapsed in the hotel room next to the room where my sister Renae and I stayed. We rushed to find hotel staff to unlock the door to her room, since my wheelchair-bound cousin, my aunt's daughter, couldn't reach the door latch to let us in. Once inside, Renae started CPR. Helpless, I held my frantic cousin.

In that thin place where heaven and earth touch like a transparent piece of vellum,[3] we prayed desperate prayers. If we could have observed, we would have seen my aunt sitting on the brink of eternity, but we, being earthbound, fought so hard, so hard, to keep her with us.

Once the paramedics stabilized her heartbeat, they wheeled my aunt into an ambulance. The small-town hospital staff assessed the damage from the brain aneurism that caused my aunt to collapse and helicoptered her to the closest large city. Chance of survival? Zero.

At the hospital, a palliative care nurse went over information and told us how my aunt would receive care to make her comfortable until the family made further decisions. Several people asked questions and then the nurse turned to my cousin.

"Do you have any questions?" the nurse asked.

My cousin began to cry. "I have lots of questions, but . . ." She sobbed. She waved her hands in the air. Gasped for control.

"But what?" the nurse prompted.

"I have lots of questions, but you can't answer them," my cousin choked. "Only God can answer them."

I pull off my sweatpants, fold them neatly, and stack them on top of my shoes. I unbutton my loose-fitting blue blouse and add it to the pile, obeying the presurgery requirements of having comfortable clothing for the trip home. I stand shivering in my bra and panties, reflecting on the last time I was in the hospital—for the birth of our youngest, fourteen years ago. I was nervous that day too, of the uncertainties of childbirth, but knew the joy of holding our little son would make it worth it. I feel none of that anticipation today.

I take off my undergarments quickly, not knowing when a helpful nurse will appear unannounced. With the bra topping the stack, I shove my clothing inside a personal belongings bag. I slip my arms into the paisley blue hospital gown with the words *Property of the Hospital* stamped on the hemline. I wonder at the wording. *Who would want to take this home?*

The words only confirm my sense of dread—that I folded the last little piece of myself, stuffed it into a bag, and now belong to the hospital. Moments ago, in the admissions office, I signed a consent form stating I was aware I could die from the surgery or suffer permanent brain damage from the anesthesia.

I am no longer in control. I hate the feeling.

"I'm ready," I say, as I crawl into the bed, but I know it is a lie.

My husband and oldest daughter, Aleah, duck around the curtain. We make small talk as the medical staff takes vital signs and the breast surgeon comes in and asks if I have any other questions.

"No," I say, knowing the doctor has no answers beyond the surgery. I wonder what he would do if I let spill the dam.

21

Will I live to see all my children grow up and be married? Did I survive late-night feedings, the terrible twos, and the awkward junior high years in vain? Will I live to see the adult human beings each will become?

Will I ever hold a grandchild? Will I live to grow old and gray beside my husband? Years from now, will I reach out in the darkness and find him breathing beside me? Will we take wish-list trips to Italy and Peru? Will I hike the ruins of Machu Picchu?

Will the scar be hideous? Will the anesthesia make me nauseated? Will they cut out all the cancer? Will my husband still think I am beautiful?

The questions rage as a nurse pokes a vein for an IV, a tiny bead of blood forming near the puncture. My hands start to shake. The nurse brings in a heated hospital blanket and unfurls the blanket in one smooth motion. Kevin tucks it around me. I lean back and close my eyes. The blanket warms like the desert sun. My shivers subside as the heat seeps into my bones.

Author and naturalist Ann Haymond Zwinger writes, "Deserts are beginnings, perhaps because there are so many questions in a desert. Questions are beginnings, answers are endings, and in the desert all the answers come in the form of more questions."[4]

"Why did you bring us out to the desert to die?" the Israelites asked Moses.

"I have lots of questions, but you can't answer them," my cousin said.

In this wrestling-questioning-wandering place, one question looms paramount as I am wheeled down the hall and into the operating room: "Where is the God who answers questions?"

I am met with silence.

When the shivers return, I cannot stop them.

Two

Stupid Strong

The stitches have finally dissolved.

My fingers rub against the side of my right breast as I adjust the straps on my swimsuit. Although several weeks have gone by, I am still struggling to accept the reality of the diagnosis. I am not sure I should be swimming, but I decide not to ask so I can't be told no.

Most of the lap lanes are occupied. Two white-haired ladies with wrinkles spilling out of their spandex stretch in lanes one and two. A young guy wearing a navy Speedo churns out the laps in lane three. That leaves lane four.

Chlorine hangs in the air, stinging my eyes. My hands shake as I pull on a pair of racing goggles and fit them snuggly to my face. I will my fingers to be still.

"It's nothing," I tell myself. I shake out my hands and take cleansing breaths. I will not work myself into a panic. "It's nothing," I repeat as I push off the wall in the shallow end and dive under the cool water. My arms slice through the water with memorized rhythm as I shoot up and down the lane. I am not the best swimmer, but I am determined to get in one workout before my next surgery. The margins from the tissue removed in the last surgery did not come back clean. The doctor needs to go back and take more.

Cancer. I hate the word. *Cancer my plans. Cancer my future. Cancer my life.*

Faster and faster I push my body until my heart strains against my ribs.

I sense more than hear a swimmer come behind me in the lane. I glance through my dark goggles. Ms. Red Swimsuit. I don't know her name, but I know Red is faster than I am in the freestyle, which, to be honest, isn't saying much. But I make a decision.

You will not beat me today. I pick up my pace as Red passes me. I edge closer, finding the churn of the other woman's wake. Moving forward, my body enters her draft. *I'll conserve my energy and pass you on the final stretch.* I swim behind her feet. My body feels strong and responsive; I am in the zone. We swim one length and then another.

After swimming two hundred meters, I notice a twinge of pain under my right armpit. I adjust my arm stroke but choose to ignore it, focusing instead on pushing my legs harder in the water. My thigh muscles respond to my willpower. *I come from a long line of strong women. I can do this.* Even as Red picks up the pace, I have no trouble matching her stroke for stroke.

On the final turn, I push hard off the concrete wall. Pure, intoxicating adrenaline courses in my veins as I drive my body. At the center of the pool I pull next to Red. My lungs scream for me to stop, but I only push harder. A quick underwater glance confirms my stretched fingertips touch the wall first. *Yes! I win!*

Resting on the pool edge, I suck in air. Red continues swimming, oblivious to my accomplishment. As I reach to remove my goggles, a twinge of pain radiates up my right side. I massage the skin by my breast. The scar is sensitive. It feels like trouble.

I flip my body over for my cooldown lap—the elementary back-stroke. "Chicken-star-rocket," I whisper, repeating the words the swim instructor used to teach me the stroke when I was eight years old. My hair floats in silent strands against my cheeks.

I breathe and watch the ceiling go by, down one length and back. *Chicken-star-rocket. Chicken-star-rocket.* Usually I am able to let my negative thoughts sink to the bottom of the pool, where they can be absorbed by the chlorine. But not today. With each beat of my heart, as much as I try, I cannot erase the fact that I am facing another surgery.

Without thinking, I break my stroke to rub the scar. I remember being teased in eighth grade for not needing to wear a bra. I remember my first bikini—pink—and unfastening the clasp as I sunbathed so I wouldn't get a weird tan line. I remember my honeymoon night and later breastfeeding four children. I remember when my breasts brought pleasure and delight and fed a baby. I remember when my breasts weren't trying to kill me.[1]

I begin another lap. I concentrate on my heartbeat as it slows. One word refuses to drown.

Can-cer. Can-cer. Can-cer.

My husband's fingers follow the water droplets on my skin, chasing the moisture down to the towel edge. I wrap the towel tighter and grasp it firmly under my armpits as I turn my back on the invitation in order to inspect the closet.

"I need to go shopping," I say. I sort through hangers and dismiss first one outfit and then another. "I need looser clothes."

He sighs. Deep. And drops his hands. "How is your skin?" he asks. The question stings, for in the past he would know. Before the hiding. The surgery. The excuses. Before getting dressed in the dark. And undressed.

"My skin is burned. Raw from radiation," I admit. I peer over my shoulder to see his face.

"Are you using the special lotion?" he asks.

"Yes. Every day."

He reaches to touch me but changes his mind. I sense, more than see, the distance between us widen. "Does it bother you?" he asks.

"Does what bother me?"

"Undressing for other men."

"They're my doctors." The question surprises me. Where had it come from?

"I just wondered. Does it bother you?"

I know he is trying to figure things out in his male brain. Figure me out. I wish I could help him.

As I riffle through the clothes in the closet, his question lingers in the room. I am five weeks into the prescribed seven weeks of daily radiation treatments. Each day I disrobe for strangers, putting on a dingy blue-and-white gown with ties in unhelpful places. The garment gaps no matter how much I twist and turn in an attempt to keep myself covered.

The treatments are in a room with a hazard warning on the door: *CAUTION! High Radiation Area.* I untie my robe and lie down on the sheeted table. Professional hands use the three tiny tattoos on my skin as a guide to maneuver me in the exact position, like crosshairs on a target. I debated posting on social media, "Hey! I got my first tattoo!" but realized people would ask for a photo and changed my mind.

As a child, I enjoyed playing Battleship, a game my family received one Christmas. My brother offered to play with me after we had opened the gifts. Surrounded by boxes and ripped wrapping paper, I hid my five ships on the game's 10 × 10 grid. I placed the aircraft carrier, submarine, and cruiser near the top of the board and the two-holed destroyer in the bottom right-hand corner. The battleship I placed directly in the center. The directions explained the object of the game was to be the first player to find and sink all the opponent's ships.

"A-6."

I won that first game against my brother.

"A-4."

But now, rather than me scanning a board game for enemy ships, doctors are searching my body for something more sinister, something that has invaded it. I pray my battleship hasn't already sunk.

"You are lucky," they say. "Your cancer was detected early." *Lucky?* I hesitate to call it *my cancer*. Is it mine? Do I want to claim ownership? "At least you don't need chemo," they say. *At least? When did this become a competition?*

"Take shallow breaths," the nurse reminds me before each radiation treatment, before disappearing from the room. I try not to focus on the fact that the room is too dangerous for healthy people, that I am the only one allowed to remain. I force away images of nuclear bombs and radiation poisoning. The machine hums. I lie bare. Exposed. The radiation beats down with no place to escape.

I am a woman, not a disease. My husband touches my shoulder. My attention jolts back to him, to a closet full of clothes that rub against my raw skin.

Does it bother me to have strangers stare clinically at my bare breasts every day? One healthy. One scarred. Puckered pink on damaged skin.

My husband's eyes are on me, peering down, leaving me with no place to run. Why is the "two becoming one" so difficult even now, after many years of marriage? What is this war inside me that wants to be strong, to do it on my own? To not admit my need?

Shade awaits me, but I step back, into cloudless sun.

"It doesn't bother me," I say, my eyes on his feet. The towel clutched in fisted hands.

I choose half of two, which is different than becoming one.

I stand alone.

"Your great-great-great grandmother, Brita Gjertsdatter, sailed on the *Victor Emanuel* in 1866. She left Norway with thirty-three family members, twenty-five of whom were children." Mom tells me the story as we page through a family photo album. "When

Brita's son, Gjert, who had lived with her in the family home, decided to join his sisters, Anna and Brynhilda, in the voyage to America, Brita packed her trunk and left her beloved fjords."

"Twenty-five children! Across an ocean? I can't imagine," I say. I have heard the story before, but it is still difficult for me to wrap my brain around the details.

"Three were brand-new babies, less than four months old."

I shake my head in wonderment. What did they do for diapers on the six-week crossing?

"Brita was sixty-six years old," Mom continues. "She never wanted to leave Norway but couldn't imagine life on the family farm without her children and grandchildren."

I trace my finger down the list of names. Brita Gjertsdatter Lande. Christine Asbjornsdatter Lande. The names roll uneasily off my tongue, but their Norwegian blood flows in my veins.

One of the first tasks the women did after arriving in America was to wash clothes in a small creek. Family history reports they were thankful to God for the opportunity to start over in a new land.

Strong women. The strength of women in my family is a part of our family history; women who forged their destinies and raised their families in the face of difficult circumstances.

Brita passed on her strength to my great-great grandmother Christine, who passed the legacy to Brynhild. Brynhild's daughter, Lillian—my grandmother—married a widower with eight children. Lillian brought a young niece into the union and then they had three more children—all raised in a small two-bedroom farmhouse where one spring the mud piled so thick, my mom remembers first taking a garden hoe to the kitchen floor before mopping.

Brita to Christine to Brynhild to Lillian to Mom to me. Six generations of women of incredible strength who lived a legacy of faith and family. Women with a tendency to roll up their shirtsleeves and do what needed to be done without much fuss and bother.

From them I learned how to be strong, yet somewhere the message got twisted. I equated strength with not needing help. Like the

Israelites, I thought I could make it on my own. When faced with a God who did not answer my questions, I sought my own answers.

Why did you bring me out to the desert to die?

The question continues to pursue me. I ask the question—on examining tables. In doctors' offices. Alone in the bathroom at 2:00 a.m. *Why did you bring me out to the desert to die?* Why? Why?

The *why* question swirls and my fist shakes heavenward, but my heart whispers another question. *Who? Who are you, God?*

It is not a question of power, but a question of relationship. And isn't this the question we all murmur in dark places?

I know He can heal, but will He heal me? I know He is love, but does He love me? Will He encounter me in the sand, in the heat, in the barrenness? Who is God, really?

Perhaps it has nothing to do with my strong Norwegian blood, but instead it has to do with my human blood that begs me to ask the questions—questions murmured in a garden, "Did God really say . . . ?" Choices are made and my own hand reaches for the fruit, because don't I also want to be like God? Don't I want to *be* God? Through the ages, isn't this what haunts us—the wanting to be strong and the discovering we are not? The fist clenching for control as everything normal slips through our grasp? The answer only found in the *Who*—in the Someone beyond ourselves?

Until I find the answer to this question, I cannot answer the question I see reflected in my husband's eyes as I attempt to be strong under the desert sun. I lie stripped bare and naked. My *whys* must become *who* as I search for something . . . or rather, Someone . . . to cover me as my own strength trembles.

Three

When Theology
Has No Handhold

"Are you sure we aren't lost?" I ask as we stumble down an endless trail of sage and prickly pear cactus.[1] The last trail marker was about two miles back.

"We will turn left at the base of that next ridgeline," Kevin says. "About a half mile later we will reach the fork in the trail. We will turn right and make our way back to our car."

It is not unusual for my husband to scrutinize landmarks in the desert to determine where we are and where we are heading. What is unusual is for him to be turned around. He carries an internal compass that is rarely confused. As for me, the ridgelines, hills, and mountains morph into one solid mass in my mind. I can identify nothing.

The hike began five hours earlier, a 9.2-mile loop in the Superstition Mountains starting at First Water Trailhead. Rather than racing quickly through the wilderness, the wildflowers beckoned us to stop often to take pictures. Pink fairyduster, Indian paintbrush, tiny blue dicks, lupines, and yellow and orange desert rock peas are only a few of the plants in full bloom.

Small purple butterflies lured Mollie into romps around the brittlebush, the golden flowers moving softly in the slight breeze. A close brush with a teddy bear cholla brought a yelp and a pause, as Mollie lifted the injured paw and waited for us to remove the clump of cactus with a pair of pliers before she bounded off on more adventures.

At the juncture of Black Mesa and Dutchman Trails, we stopped to take photographs of Weaver's Needle, a prominent one-thousand-foot spire left over from an eroded volcano. Somewhere we made a wrong turn among the various washes.

I repeat my question, "Are you sure we are not lost?" The Needle is in front of us when it should be behind us. "Are there two needles?"

"Only one," Kevin says. "We got turned around."

"Are you sure?"

He pulls out a compass, a device that is a complete mystery to me. He hands me the topographic map and I choke on my granola bar. He knows I am directionally challenged. *North*, *south*, *east*, and *west* are only words in the dictionary in my mind. I can get turned around taking a different exit out of a neighborhood. My lack of direction is legendary.

I remember one time we got lost on vacation. Somewhere. On a cross-country road trip. In the days before GPS and cell phones and Google Maps.

My husband threw the map at me as he drove.

"Tell me where we are and where we are going," he said.

"What state are we in?" I asked. (Like I said. Legendary.)

He ground out an answer.

I thought about saying we were in the state of confusion but decided my wit would not be appreciated. I asked several other questions, turning the map so it was not upside down. The car was completely quiet; no noise came from our four children as they realized their fates had been handed to their clueless mother. I had often wondered why drive-up ATMs had Braille lettering but realized the map in my hands might as well have been in Braille for all the sense I could make of it.

Now, standing in the shade of what I am convinced is a second Weaver's Needle, I am equally clueless.

When up is down, right is left, and things that are not appear as though they are, we tell ourselves many things. Often untrue.

———

When my treatment ends, I try my best to bury it under the file of ancient history in my brain. For the first time in months, people believe me when I say I am fine, and conversations continue like everything is normal, because in their minds it is. I convince myself life is also back to precancer normal, minus the quarterly doctor appointments and daily medication to keep the dragon in the cave.

I am not fine. I find myself looking over my shoulder to find the woman who existed before cancer. She has wandered off in the distance in a landscape where ridgelines, hills, and mountains have morphed into one solid mass. I feel bewildered in familiar places. Same husband. Same house. Same kids. Same routine.

Yet everything has been turned on its head.

I am reminded of a story my parents tell of the first time Dad went to see Mom at her family's home in rural South Dakota. The final penciled directions Dad held in his hand all those decades ago were easy: *turn at the woods and take the dirt road to the farm.*

Simple.

Except my dad grew up in northern Wisconsin, where woods meant acres and acres of tall trees. Cedars. Firs. Pines. Tamaracks. Mom grew up surrounded by unending flat fields with a gathering of trees—her idea of woods—planted as a windbreak at the edge of a neighbor's property.

My dad drove past Mom's trees. He was lost, wandering around, searching for the familiar.

I can relate. I'm traveling down the post-treatment road, and I'm not sure where to turn. How did what was once so familiar change into something I no longer recognize? I find myself going as fast as I can. Normal in our family means driving a full schedule, and everyone is glad to have me back in the midst of the busy intersection directing traffic. With four children—one married, one in college, and two in high school—the calendar quickly fills with various activities. The community in which we volunteer and the congregation where we pastor consume the remaining white spaces.

It's as if I want to make up for lost time. Filling the calendar is my way of bringing control again into a life that was out of control. Six months after treatment I compete with my daughter Aleah in a triathlon, determined to run any lingering effects of cancer into the ground. I enroll in college writing classes, sitting next to students younger than my own children.

But no matter how fast I run, there is one area in which I have no control—the possibility of recurrence. I find myself distracted and easily overwhelmed. I know I should be elated that treatment is over, but I wander through my days, unsure what to do.

Are there two of me—the one who could multitask and was never flustered and the one who now freaks out at every sniffle and swollen lymph node?

"There is a lump on my face by my left ear," I inform the doctor at one of my quarterly appointments, proud that my voice is clipped and analytical, with not a speck of the worry that disrupted the past three nights of sleep.

The doctor feels the lump for two seconds. Tops. "Swollen lymph node from your sinus infection," she says. Apparently two can play the analytical game.

"Isn't it large for a lymph node?" I ask, my fingers involuntarily rubbing my skin.

The doctor looks up from her note-taking. Maybe my voice isn't as nonchalant as I imagine.

She feels my jawline again. She knows my history. She looks in my eyes and I see compassion. "If the lump is still there after you finish the antibiotic, come back and see me."

I nod numbly.

Oh Jesus, help me. Has the cancer returned? Is it in my lymph system? Will they have to cut my face?[2]

"When will life be back to normal?" I ask a friend when the lump turns out to be nothing.

She laughs. "Normal is a setting on a dryer."

I nod, because haven't I also laughed in the past at this joke? I want to scream, "This has nothing to do with dryer settings!" But I stuff the emotions down. Perhaps I can cram more into the opening, push the button, and shut the door, because isn't the winner the one who can squash in the most things?

I am lost. Lost in my own story. Is my map upside down? Or is it me?

My family and I make plans to travel to the Havasu Canyon, a remote area that requires a ten-mile hike to the campground. It's one of our favorite vacation spots, and we no longer need a map to navigate this remote wilderness of narrow canyon walls.

The beginning of the hike is steep with switchbacks winding down a rocky trail for one and a half miles. After the switchbacks, the trail curves through a narrow canyon for six and a half miles before hikers arrive at the village of Supai, home to the Havasupai—the "people of blue-green waters"—an isolated community accessible only by foot, helicopter, or mule. The campground is located an additional two miles past the village.

Of the four waterfalls that can be reached from the campground, Moonie Falls is the most difficult to explore. The trail down the sandstone cliffs meanders through a maze of narrow tunnels, rickety ladders, iron handholds, and rusted chains covered in slippery mist. My husband and I have had to call forth an inner Indiana Jones in more than one hiker who balked at the challenging obstacle course through the travertine formations.

The last time we came, our children played in the turquoise pool continuously refilled by the falls, a two-hundred-foot splurge of free-falling water. The cool water relieved stiff muscles from the long hike in the day before. Soaking blistered feet was soon not enough and invariably a dare was issued by several high schoolers: "Who wants to swim behind the falls?"

"I'm in!"

"Me too!" they shouted.

Towels were tossed aside and toes were dipped into the cold water. Kevin arched an eyebrow in my direction, but I shook my head, content in the sunbeams.

The adventurous ones—including my husband—waded first, stepping cautiously through the cool water. After a few minutes, they dove in, forced to commit. The water pulsated from all sides. Bubbles massaged their skin while continuous bucket loads dropped with unrelenting force from above, creating waves around them. The turbulence multiplied as they neared the falls.

From past experience I knew the currents twisted around arms and legs, dragging at limbs, seeking to pull people under. No longer falling in buckets, the water was one continuous sheet of force and sound. The bass notes pounded in ears. Against chests.

One solid roar.

From the shore I watched as again and again swimmers attempted to get closer to the falls, but the forceful water falling from above combined with the suction dragging them under was too much. Each adventurer turned back. No one made it behind the falls. Toweling off, they warmed themselves in a strip of sunshine.

Our family consumed our bagels and cream cheese on a lush piece of ground watered by the showering mist as we lingered in this little piece of heaven, this "Garden of Eden" in Arizona.

The trip to Havasu Canyon doesn't happen. Flash floods, a problem in the past, came again, surprising hikers and campers and wiping out portions of the trail. Even the village of Supai was damaged. Previously, the plumbing system had been destroyed and the homes had been leveled and carried downstream in one huge wall of water over the falls—Moonie Falls.

What would we do in a flash flood?

A shiver runs through me as I watch the report on the news.

I remember the only way out via narrow tunnels, a rickety ladder, iron handholds, and rusted chains—all coated in slippery mist. I try to imagine clinging to the natural handholds on the canyon walls, waiting to be rescued, while floodwaters raged below. Could I cling there for hours?

In the past, hikers have been rescued from trees, from narrow ledges, from tiny slivers of higher ground. The floodwaters lapped at their feet while they attempted to stretch one inch higher. Others died in the narrow canyon, caught in the turbulent, unforgiving water.[3]

Water in the desert kills in two ways. Not enough. Or too much.

I have always been afraid of drowning.

The first wave hits fourteen months after I finish treatment.

Cancer. My mother writes the word in a family email. "Your dad has cancer." The words swirl and twist. Is it new fear or old? I cannot decipher the difference.

"Metastatic melanoma. Stage 4."

What began as a surgery to remove a jawline cyst has spiraled into the most severe diagnosis. The most ominous.

"Cancer is a word, not a sentence," people say, but the syllables drag at me and suck—suck me down, drowning out my very breath.

I claw at canyon walls, seeking a handhold. My fingers cling to a narrow crack in the cliff face. I pull myself onto a narrow ledge.

The floodwaters roll, black and angry. Gone is the translucent turquoise water. Gone are the natural swimming pools, encapsulated by travertine ledges. Gone is the tenuous peace I found after my own cancer diagnosis and treatment.

The torrent grabs at chunks of earth and tears them free.

All I can do is hold on.

A mask is made for Dad to wear during treatment. The mask is screwed to the table to keep him immobile for the precise radiation. When the cancer moves to Dad's lungs, he qualifies for a clinical trial. Months go by. Eighteen months of one chemo drug and then another. Of highs and lows. Of flights back and forth to Minnesota.

Life has a new rhythm.

Tentatively, I inch away from my narrow ledge. I turn belly-flat into the cliff face so I can inch my body down the damp rock. A rumble to my left alerts me. Instinctively, I know. Is it possible? The noise crescendoes to a roar.

I gulp one life-saving gasp of air before the next flood wave hits.

"Cancer," Mom telephones. "I have cancer."

A biopsy comes back from a swollen lymph node from Mom's groin. Ovarian cancer. Lymph node involvement from her neck to her pelvis. Metastatic. The only treatments available are life-extending.

Both of my parents have cancer. Incurable cancer.

With my cancer diagnosis I believed I could take back everything cancer took from me. I bought into our culture's mind-set that health is the only option after sickness, even from cancer. Not only did my doctors speak the language of the healed, but I heard the words in my own mind and from the lips of my friends. But now? How do I find words for this story? Where does it fit in my narrative that "every suffering has a remedy"?[4]

I lose my grip. I tumble into floodwaters. The map I drew from my cancer journey washes away. Twisting and turning, boulders whipping around me like unmoored boats, I thrash helplessly in surging water. I have competed in triathlons; surely I can muscle my way through.

My strength fails. I have nothing. I am nothing.

My theology has no handhold for this.

"The rain fell, and the floods came, and the winds blew and slammed against that house; and it fell—and great was its fall" (Matt. 7:27).

The panic tugs me down.

I am in a desert.

I am drowning.

Where can I find solid ground? Where is my compass? My map?

My oxygen-starved brain seeks an answer. Countless sermons, prayer meetings, and Bible stories, yet I come up empty.

God is not a liar. The thought beats a steady tempo, louder than the surging floodwaters. *God is not a liar.* I don't understand much else, but I grab on to this truth.

Memorized phrases from long-ago Sunday school throw me into an eddy, a current running counter to the heaving swells. "When you go through deep waters, I will be with you. When you go through rivers of difficulty, you will not drown. . . . For I am the LORD, your God" (Isa. 43:2–3 NLT).

I will be with you. The momentary relief gives me space to reach for a tiny ledge of hope.

My arm stretches, tendons pulling. The water pounds above and around and seeks to suck me back down. I grasp the small handhold—barely deep enough for four fingers. Incredibly, my grip holds. I lift my head for an inch of breathing space.

I hold on tight in surging waters.

I will be with you.

Four

I Will Live until I Die

Mom starts chemotherapy alongside Dad—the dynamic chemo duo. The nurses say rarely do both spouses go through cancer at the same time. Dad jokes that being above average is overrated.

I live across the country. At times it is more than I can bear. The walls close in and I flee to nighttime skies. Away from closing walls. Away from closing questions.

In a nearby water retention basin, away from streetlights, I stare upward at the blackness, not just a few stars, but layers and layers, spilling over each other in the night sky.

The Big Dipper. Orion, the good hunter. The North Star. Pleiades, the Seven Sisters. The creamy expanse of the Milky Way. Thousands upon thousands of stars, which are nameless to me, but not to the One who counts their number.

I serve a God who counts. Who likes numbers.

He counts stars. He counts the hairs on a head—even on the head of a cancer patient. He holds the dimensions of the earth. He considers lilies. He watches over sparrows. The first created work He numbered was a day.

"There was evening and there was morning, one day" (Gen. 1:5). He called the light *day* and the darkness *night*. He put time

41

boundaries on His new creation and called it good. Time is a God-created idea.

After the formation of the earth, God continued to count days. He didn't use a wristwatch or a calendar. He wrote numbers in a book, before the days were in existence. "Your eyes have seen my unformed substance; and in Your book were all written the days that were ordained for me, when as yet there was not one of them" (Ps. 139:16).

Under a different nighttime sky, a man named Abraham once stood after being brought out from his tent by the hand of God to focus on the stars. Gazing into the endless expanse, God spoke to Abraham and told him to give it his best shot, to try to count the stars. Then God, the God who loves to count, spoke an incredible promise. "So shall your descendants be" (Gen. 15:5).

God took a childless man out under a desert sky and promised him an endless family tree. He spoke not only a word but a sentence—and rewrote a man's destiny.

I stand under an Arizona sky and hear whispers of my smallness. I am not childless, but I am filled with fear and doubt.

Can I trust Him? Is He big enough? Does He hear me? Does He know me?

My greatest fear is He does not know my name. Dad's name. Mom's name. Are we only numbers under a night sky?

———

I catch a flight back to the Midwest to be with my parents. My sister picks me up at the airport for the two-hour drive. As we pull into the snow-covered driveway, Dad shuffles out to help us with our luggage. Mom tries to hold her emotions together in the kitchen, but my sister hugs her neck and tells her she doesn't have to be strong. The linoleum gets wet with more than melted snow.

One step into my childhood bedroom sends me traveling back in time. I hang clothes in my tiny closet that slopes to fit the shape of the eastern roof. I recall races down the stairs with my brother and two sisters. I remember six people sharing one bathroom.

I feel young and old again. All at the same time.

Comfort finds me in the remembering, but there is no going back in time. Only forward. Dad's clothes droop off his frame. Mom wears a scarf over her bald head, but Dad still calls her "babe" and "my beautiful bride." Sitting in the living room with Dad and Mom, I have this sense that time is running out, that we are running toward a finish line I don't want to cross.

I want more time.

I. Want. More.

More afternoons of Dad doing Sudoku puzzles while Mom fixes lunch in the kitchen. More Ole and Lena jokes—Dad's favorite Norwegian pranksters. More family gatherings. More vacations with grandchildren rolling scooters down the hill. More weekly emails from Mom about relatives, projects around the property, and life in a small town. More prayers from the lips of my parents for their children and grandchildren.

We sit down for supper around the dining room table. Hands extend. Fingers grasp. Dad reaches his hand for Mom's. He grips the finger where he placed a ring fifty-five years ago.

They met while working at their college's cafeteria—she a South Dakota farm girl, he a dairy farmer's son from Wisconsin. Mom served the fruit, while Dad scooped the ice cream. "It's been peaches and cream ever since," Dad frequently quips. Now, four kids, thirteen grandchildren, five great-grandchildren, a paid-off mortgage, and five decades of memories later, they share cancer.

We bow our heads to say grace and give thanks for the evening meal. Dad forgets to pray for the food but does not forget to thank God that He is in control even on hard days.

God is in control?

After supper Mom types an email to tell family and friends about the latest developments. I have been the recipient of count-less of these informative and positive emails, but tonight I watch my mom stare at the screen and wipe her eyes. How do you find words to describe the indescribable?

We sit on the couch to watch TV. Dad pretends to watch Vanna and the spinning wheel, but in reality, his gaze rarely leaves the woman he has loved for more than half a century. He attempts to absorb the fact that they are both fighting the same dragon. He has pledged for better and for worse, in sickness and in health, and this is where the vow has brought them.

Disturbed, I go to the kitchen to make a cup of tea. As I place the mug in the microwave, my finger pauses over a control button: "Add 30 Seconds." Right there. Under the number nine. A button I have never noticed before.

Add 30 Seconds.

I'd like to yank the button off the microwave and stick it to my life. Our lives. And not to minor items like the dashboard of my car so when the stoplight turns yellow, I can hit the button and sail through the intersection. As much as I'd like to add it to my morning schedule when chaos reigns as our youngest tries to get out to marching band practice before the sun rises, I would not waste the button there.

I spent Katelyn's senior year traveling back and forth with Dad's cancer. It appears I will spend Zach's senior year doing more of the same, but with Mom added. I am tempted to put a button on Zach's forehead to slow down the upcoming year of *lasts*. Last band concert. Last award ceremony. Last day of classes. As much as I am tempted, I am aware that to place the button on my son would make his world smaller, not larger. I have raised him to enter a world of his making, not mine. The microwave beeps. Heated mug in hand, I stand by the large picture windows in my parents' living room. I trace my finger along the finished oak trim. This. This is where I'd like to place the button, so when Mom gazes out at the neighboring fields, she can give the button a tap. Every evening, when Dad makes one more round to make sure each door and window is locked, he can push the button.

While I stand here, I can push the button once. Or twice. Or a thousand times.

I stare at the night sky—of stars that spill out on winter-covered ground. The Big Dipper. Orion. The North Star. I have flown halfway across the country, but when I look up, I am home. I traveled many miles, but under the heavens, I am, essentially, exactly where I was before.

The silence wraps around me, swallowing me in its embrace, until I swear I can hear the silence speak. Psalm 147:4–5 echoes, "He counts the number of the stars; He gives names to all of them. Great is our Lord and abundant in strength; His understanding is infinite."

I am small, but I hear another message in the night air.

You are not forgotten.

It's that type of night. A night for hearing the present voice of God as I stand desperate. A night for discovering the bigness of God—the hugeness of a counting God who does not treat me like a number but who knows my name. He, who names the stars, calls my name.

"Do not be afraid . . . I have called you by name; you are mine" (Isa. 43:1 NLT). I belong to Him. To be named is the first basic element of a person's identity. A symbol of welcome. Of belonging. Of family. Of arriving home.

Home to Albert Lea, Minnesota. Home to my childhood house. Home to the shade of God. Is it possible?

I hear the truth under starry skies. I want more time, but *more* is never satisfied. More has no definable boundaries, so it is never full. We push, pull, drive, and squeeze time seeking *more*. Thirty *more* seconds. But *more* runs ahead of us. Always. Right beyond our grasp. *More* is not a word for this side of life.

It is not a word for "there was evening and there was morning, one day" (Gen. 1:5). More is a word for eternity.

I force myself to face the question. How many additional thirty seconds do I want?

If Dad lives three more years, will it be enough time? No. If Mom lives five years? Still not enough. How about fifteen? Will that be enough time? No. Absolutely not. Everything in my daughter-heart rebels at the thought of losing my dad. My mom. At any age. My heart tells me there has to be more to life than this.

All hearts whisper the same words. We were created for a place without time.

C. S. Lewis wrote, "Creatures are not born with desires unless satisfaction for those desires exists. A baby feels hunger: well, there is such a thing as food. A duckling wants to swim: well, there is such a thing as water. . . . If I find myself a desire which no experience in this world can satisfy, the most probable explanation is that I was made for another world."[1]

Dad puts it into perspective when he says, "I will live until I die, and then my real life will begin." He repeats it frequently, every time someone asks how he is doing. "I will live until I die, and then my real life will begin."

I can't argue with that logic. That faith. That truth.

I hear the whisper from the Maker of the stars that my parents' world is about to get larger, not smaller. My desire to install an "Add 30 Seconds" button to their lives would prevent them from moving into their next chapters. To keep them here would be in a world of my making, not God's.

Around Mom's name, around Dad's name, around my name, God has set a boundary to our days. He counts the days and calls them good. This is love in action. A God who loves me. Mom. Dad. You. Who created limits, but limits with a name. We are known. Each day we move closer to timelessness. Forever. Eternity. More.

God who lives in a place of timelessness, a boundaryless place of more, has written those days in a book. Some have one page. Some have one hundred pages. But in each and every heart, He has placed the promise of a life beyond this life.

We cannot forget.

If we run and hope for more in any other place but in eternity, we will be desolate. Angry. Ragged. No matter how much we love, if we believe we have forever here on earth, we will set ourselves up for inconsolable agony. We must ponder the night skies and remember, especially on days we are most afraid.

> Star Namer
> World Spinner
> When the depth of my fear overwhelms me
> Help me remember
> That if you can count the number of stars
> And be on a first-name basis
> With each one
> Then you are Big Enough
> You are Big Enough.

God, who loves numbers, invites me to stand with Him under the shade of time. He calls my name and I understand something about this number-loving God.

His favorite number is one.

Five

Allee, Allee, All Come Free

My husband and I get up at 4:00 a.m. to make the drive to Sycamore Canyon in Arizona for a morning of hiking. The day is perfect. Low humidity. Temperature in the high 70s. We hope to beat the crowds of those who come to this area of Arizona to experience the contrast in color—the lush green by the stream versus the unique mix of the rock layers that frame this area—the dark basalt, red sandstone, and cream limestone.

We also come for the contrast in temperatures from the oven where we live. This is usually a high-traffic trail, but we meet only one other family on the first half of a seven-mile loop that crosses the streambed six times.

We lunch by a stream-fed pool where the sun has not yet appeared to sizzle the water. Water bugs dance on the surface, leaving tiny ripple circles, but other than that, the pool is silent. A bosk of mesquite trees—a woodland—creates a barrier for this riparian area that separates us from the harsh desert in the distance, luring us to believe in days without a thorn.

An otter—the first we've seen in the wild—pokes his head around the watercress. We hope for a photo, but the little fellow is camera shy. The otter dives and swims among the shadows, finally returning to his hiding place along the shore.

After our snack of apples and string cheese, Mollie is glad to return to her side adventures of crouching low to chase butterflies and lizards into the underbrush. The lizards scamper so quickly to their hiding spaces in the rock crevices that I have no opportunity to name them.

Mollie is the first to sense the danger.

Unsure, she backs into Kevin's legs.

Camouflaged by its dusty gray and brown diamond-shaped markings, a diamondback rattlesnake lies coiled on the trail, shaking his rattle, unhappy to be interrupted from his morning dose of sunlight. Kevin grabs Mollie's collar.

We freeze. Kevin asks for the camera and gives Mollie to me. The three-foot snake coils tighter. We count eight segments on the rattle—one for each time the snake has shed its skin—still shaking in warning. On the tail, above the rattle, we notice the white and black bands, distinctive to all western diamondbacks. We don't know if the snake has left his shelter to warm his cold-blooded body or to seek a meal. We know one thing—we don't want to be mistaken for a snack.

"Remember, snakes can strike the length of their body," I say, as my husband moves in for a closer photograph. Kevin takes a step back.

"I need to move the snake," he says after several photos. "That family is still behind us." I remember the two preteen kids with their mom and dad. They were more focused on fishing in the stream than searching for poisonous reptiles.

"Don't become a statistic," I caution.

"Not planning on it," Kevin says as he gets a long stick to poke the snake. He knows as well as I do that a woman will most likely be bitten on the ankle or leg when she unwittingly steps too close to a rattler, but a guy will usually be bitten on the arm or hand after messing with the snake. We have joked about it in the past.

The snake shakes its rattle harder and raises its triangular head in a tighter coil. Its black tongue flickers. The snake has claimed ownership to this particular section of trail and has no intention of budging from his little kingdom.

Kevin tries again. Same result.

Finally he snags a section of the snake with the stick and lifts it. The snake writhes, unhappy with this turn of events, evicted from his place of residence. Once down, the rattler slithers into the bushes, through some leaves, and under a rock. Safely hidden.

The desert is a good place for hiding.

———

"Allee, allee, all come free."

The words echoed across the three acres on which sat my childhood home. I burrowed deeper under the honeysuckles, wiggling to get my tanned nine-year-old legs under the poky branches. I imagined myself to be invisible so my siblings and friends could not find me.

"Allee, allee, all come free!"

The call came again for everyone who was still hiding to come out into the open without penalty of losing the game. My younger sister was "it," and I had watched her find friends hiding in the barn, in the pine tree, and behind the garden shed. I wondered if I was the only one left hiding.

A mosquito buzzed near my ear and I shooed it away. It was the only sound in the now silent backyard. I pushed a branch aside and peeked out.

Where was everyone? Had they gone to play with the new kittens in the haymow? Were they getting a snack in the kitchen? Had they moved on to a game at someone else's house?

I army-crawled out from the hedge and stood up. Slowly. I didn't want to give away my great hiding spot, for I planned to use it again. I walked past the teeter-totter and swings. I peered cautiously around the corner of the one-car garage, sliding spread eagle against the rough, white-painted wood. I heard voices by the garden.

My sister swung a mallet and her orange ball went rolling toward a wicket set on the far edge of the lawn by the culvert. The ball hopped over a clump of clover and stopped inches from someone's yellow ball. They had started a game of croquet without me!

I sauntered down, a touch of bravado in my voice, teasing them for giving up so quickly. A neighborhood friend twirled her mallet, taking off the heads of two dandelions. She pointed her mallet at me, like a sword.

"The point of the game is to be found," she said.

"Can you give an update at church about your parents?" my husband asks as I lean close to the bathroom mirror to put on mascara one Sunday morning.

"Sure," I say, nodding. Confident. How hard can one short announcement be? I've been giving them for weeks.

Several hours later I stand with the intention of giving a word-for-word report: Mom bumped her head getting into the car the day before and was blinded in her eye for five minutes. The doctor, calling it a ministroke, was concerned.

I open my mouth to give the intended report but am suddenly speechless. Since my diagnosis, I have embraced the language of the healed, of the victorious, of the strong, of kicking cancer in the teeth. I have no words for this story.

Only tears. A few trickle down in black streaks, followed by gut-wrenching sobs from a hidden place no longer content to be silenced.

My storm cloud bursts. I am undone.

Mom's diagnosis, following so quickly after Dad's, has caused my tears to flow uncontrollably in public and often when I least expect it. I cry on the airplane. In the car. Next to the organic zucchini in the grocery store. Bent over the computer as I pray for a key to backspace my life.

At Olive Garden, tears land in my bowl of Zuppa Toscana. Grief finds a home in the cream and kale and sausage while an attentive waiter keeps bringing more bread sticks.

Cancer has robbed me of my ability to hide, a skill I learned from childhood. A skill perhaps also carried in my blood, from back when my ancestors hid in bushes at the cool of the day and God came seeking them, asking, "Where are you?"[1]

"Illness is about learning to live with lost control,"[2] author Arthur W. Frank writes in *The Wounded Storyteller.* Whenever Mom sends a new email or calls with another report from the doctor, I find myself processing first on an analytical level, finding comfort in the medical terminology. But the utter chaos of my parents' combined story has torn away all illusion of control. I barely process one layer of loss before another assault rips the ground away beneath my feet.

We live in a society where one of the current challenges is to *be present.* We are urged to turn off our cell phones and put down the cameras and stop posting minute-by-minute updates on social media in an effort to be known. It is one thing to be present in the moments of happy milestone events like concerts, birthday parties, weddings, and graduations. It is another to be present in the moments of the difficult, to step out of hiding into a non-Photoshopped life.

What if the now finds me facing my greatest fear? Can I truly be present in that reality? Even in the broken? The messy? The out-of-controlness of loss?

Jesus calls Himself *I Am.* He promises to be present in the engulfing helplessness of this current moment.

I know this is the strength I must run to. I must leave behind the false shade and stand exposed. My faith says here I will discover foundness. Yet, what does this even mean?

"Where can I go from your Spirit? Where can I flee from your presence? If I go up to the heavens, you are there; if I make my bed in the depths, you are there" (Ps. 139:7–8 NIV).

Oh, the irony!

Tallest mountain. Driest desert. Deepest valley. There is no place to hide from God, but once naked and bare, He invites me to hide myself in Him.

Vulnerable. Messy. Afraid. The point is to be found.

Allee, allee, all come free.

Six

Love in the Bending Low

Although rain is in the forecast, Kevin and I decide to drive one hundred miles for a picnic lunch. We see no evidence of clouds on the horizon as we head north out of Payson on Highway 87. We turn left at the sign for Tonto Natural Bridge and drive down the 14 percent grade on a serpentine road until we get to the ranger station. We park the car and grab our backpacks, hitting the Pine Creek Trail. A raven caws overhead as we palm hot boulders almost too warm to touch in the creek bed.

We follow the dry creek into the hollow that is the longest natural travertine bridge in the world. We are dwarfed under the rising arch, a 440-foot-long tunnel that measures 150 feet at the widest point.[1]

We pass families unprepared for a walk under the travertine. A man lugs around water in an awkward one-gallon jug. A teen, wearing flip-flops, juggles a backpack, plus a full shoulder bag. Another scrambles over the rocks with a pink cell phone, although this area has no reception. Several families carry babies in their arms—without child carriers.

Why do they come? Why leave couches in comfortable homes? Why leave air-conditioned vehicles to go tramping among the boulders with a real risk of falling?

Why? Because the desert has been 124 days without rain—124 days! Hearts are barren, parched, and thirsty for water.

So they come. So we come.

Not to an ocean. Not to a lake. Not to a river. No, to a tiny creek bed that unfolds into a cavernous space. To a travertine ceiling that drips water. Not gushes. Not flows. Drips.

Drop by precious drop.

We pull out bagels and cream cheese for a picnic on a boulder. I separate the M&Ms from the trail mix and pop the circles of chocolate in my mouth one by one.

Water falls from 183 feet above us, landing as cold polka dots on legs and shoulders. The drops fall in a continuous game of follow-the-leader before joining the other skydivers in a collective pool, their liquid feet forming growing circles in the water. A warm breeze catches the drops, swirling them in a dance of sunlight.

Captured light in water.

I stand mesmerized at the falling moisture, drops like fire opals emblazoned by sun. A jeweler's facets are nothing compared to the colors that blink for less than a second. Translucent orange. Blue. Green.

I can't help but remember a day when my husband would have done anything for a few drops of water.

Several years ago Kevin and five other cyclists headed out for a training ride. Needing to put some miles on their legs for an upcoming triathlon, they chose a forty-five-mile course along the Salt River, a barren stretch with little vegetation and fewer houses. The plan was to finish the workout before the temperatures peaked at a predicted 104 degrees.

The ride did not go as planned.

A new rider slowed the group's cadence. Three flat tires, each taking fifteen to twenty minutes to change, jeopardized the schedule. As the sun rose higher, the level in water bottles on bike frames sank lower. Lips chapped as salt dried on cracked skin. Spit turned thick and pasty.

Stopping for one more flat tire, the group accessed their water supply. The new rider's containers were empty.

Before water could be shared, a car pulling a flatbed trailer sped past. The driver ignored the cyclists on the shoulder and the riders were too surprised to flag him down. The vehicle took the curve too fast, causing a Styrofoam cooler in the back of the trailer to bounce out, shattering as it hit the asphalt.

The contents spilled, practically in slow motion, at the cyclists' feet. Gatorade, bottled water, juices, and ice littered the roadway as the vehicle raced off into the distance.

Easy water.

———

The desert is not usually a place of spilling water. Under the natural bridge, we shoulder our packs and climb to the rim. Glancing at the horizon, our eyes fix on a cloud-filled sky holding the promise of rain. Gray has never looked more beautiful.

The time of winter rains has begun, bringing a season of easy water—an oasis of time we have not enjoyed since Mom's and Dad's diagnoses. Chemo barely slows down Mom's speed of life as she organizes both of their doctors' appointments with charts, calendars, and a medical folder thick with new priorities.

The clinical trial proves effective. The tumors in Dad's lungs shrink by 50 percent, along with a majority of the other patients' tumors in the trial. Dad's oncologist, who has buried patients for twenty-five years, speaks words of a possible breakthrough.

We wonder in careful corners. *Is a cure possible? Is it a miracle?* We gather drops of hope in our collective heart pools.

The winter also brings the planning of a wedding for our daughter Aleah. With the planning comes the list. Not any old list, but The Very Detailed, Organized, Impressive Wedding To-Do List—a six-page document of details for an outdoor ceremony. The list begins as an orderly, typed stack of papers but soon morphs into a hodgepodge of scribbled notes in all the margins with many exclamation points: "Talk to the DJ about the order of music!" "Go over schedule with the park decorator!" "Get ladders!!!!"

A wedding is all about the details. When I ask Aleah to prioritize the list, she writes one item at the top of the first page, in large letters: TREES.

Yes, trees. My daughter's first priority is to have a wedding under the trees. Now, trees would not be difficult if we lived in Minnesota or Colorado or California, but we live in the Sonoran Desert, where cactus is more prevalent than maples, and many people place rocks in their front yards rather than grass. Under the blazing 115-degree summer heat, many plants wither and die no matter how hard a person tries. In Arizona, trees are a luxury item.

Thankfully, we discover a nearby park that allows weddings under decades-old branches, trees that have withstood years of monsoon winds and blistering desert summers. Our daughter decides it is a good place to put down beginning roots for a marriage.

Dad and Mom fly out ten days before the wedding. When they walk out of the gate at the airport, I rush to hug Mom, and then Dad, but I am not sure who holds the other person tighter. Dad calls me his favorite daughter, but I know if my sisters were here, they would each be his favorite also.

He draws out the word *fav . . . o . . . rite*, so my heart hears the truth-words in each syllable, drop by drop.

"What can I do?" Dad asks the next morning as we women sit at the kitchen table going over the few remaining items on The List.

"I need signs made so people know where to park," I say. "The area can be confusing."

"I can do that," Dad says.

I give Dad the supplies and move on to other tasks.

"Where's Dad?" I ask several hours later.

"He's still making wedding signs," Mom says from the sink, where she is doing the dishes.

"Still?" I step out on the back porch where Dad is bending over a piece of white poster board. A stack of finished signs leans against the table leg. "Can I get you some iced tea?"

Dad doesn't even look up. "Nope. Almost done."

I watch from the doorway as he marks letters using a template that he hand cut with meticulous care. While I would have scribbled a few lines on the poster board with a black marker, Dad carefully traces and fills in each letter. At the bottom he adds an arrow to point the way.

When I was younger, I thought love was the romantic, happily-ever-after experience I read about in books or saw on the movie screen. I thought it came with flowers and chocolate and pleasant background music. I didn't understand love is sometimes spoken without words.

Love is in the details. Love is found in the bending over. The stooping low. The care shown for the small things.

Jesus had a thing for crumbs.

In the story of feeding the five thousand, Jesus not only cared about hungry people, but he also cared about crumbs. "And they all ate and were satisfied. They picked up what was left over of the broken pieces, twelve full baskets" (Matt. 14:20).

Why did Jesus have the disciples pick up the leftovers?

Were there antilittering laws in place and Jesus didn't want his disciples to get in trouble? Or were the leftovers for the poor? Maybe they were going to drop them off at a food bank on the way home.

Why didn't they leave the crumbs for the birds?

Perhaps Jesus knew what I know—disciples tend to have soul amnesia. In the dark hours, miracles are forgotten, and in this case, the miracle had been consumed. No formerly blind person was left walking around with perfect eyesight. No lame person was giving high fives. Simply a quick fast-food stop at Long John Silver's for some fish and bread, one meal in the more than one thousand meals eaten that year.

The days of hunger and thirst are not remembered in a place of easy water.

So the disciples picked up leftovers. As they stooped, bent low, and filled twelve baskets, the abundance of the miracle they had witnessed was highlighted with each crust that was rescued. When the difficult came and the easy water dried up, the disciples would not so easily forget an extravagant, abundantly providing God.

In the night watches, when the disciples couldn't sleep, when there was no food in the cupboard, they would remember the miracle and God's faithfulness. When all they had was small and unable to provide for needs that were so great, they would remember the multiplying power of God.

I am no different. I have soul amnesia, which is why I drive a hundred miles for a picnic under the travertine. I too quickly forget. I need to remember a God who is as vast as an ocean yet catches sunlight in single drops. An extravagant God who takes a small amount and multiplies it to feed a crowd but also goes after the one; a God who cares about drops, leftovers, and broken fragments.

———

One important item remains unfinished on The List—my dress for the ceremony. Oh, I have a dress. The garment hangs from a bag on my bedroom door. The just-in-case-I-can't-find-anything-else dress.

I don't love it, but I'm tired of looking. I'm tired of foo-foo dresses with too many ruffles. I'm tired of dresses blinding my eyes with bling. I'm tired of sensible, matronly dresses. I'm tired of dresses that make me look like a hooker.

In desperation, I purchased the dress that hangs on the door. When I think of it, I feel nothing. Meh.

I tell this to my husband while we run some last-minute errands at the mall.

"Let's go dress shopping," he suggests. He is suddenly a man on a mission.

"I've already spent two days trying on dresses at this mall," I say, resistant to more dressing room horrors.

"How about this store?" he asks, pointing to a shop on the left.

"Too expensive."

"Let's go see what they have."

I hesitate.

"You should feel beautiful at our daughter's wedding," he says.

So that is how I find myself in a dressing room, with a very helpful attendant and six dresses. I set down my purse and kick off my shoes. *What just happened here? I have been married to this man for more than thirty years, and he has never, ever, gone dress shopping with me.*

Some miracles have nothing to do with clinical trials.

The first dress won't zip up and clings to my hips, showing every imperfection. I slip out of it and make vows to return to the gym and do the stair stepper every single day for a month. I reach for the second dress. I adjust the fabric as the soft material unfolds over my skin. I turn toward the floor-length mirror and catch my breath.

The dress is lovely. Not too foo-foo. Not too matronly. It is just what I've been looking for.

Kevin is on the phone when I step out of the dressing room in the midnight blue, floor-length gown. "Just a minute," he says to the person on the other end, "a gorgeous woman is modeling a dress for me."

I twirl so he can see the back. I remember walking down the aisle in another dress, confident in the approval I would find in his eyes. More than thirty years later, after breast cancer and some extra pounds, I am not so confident. The drought of cancer has sucked more than my body dry, as we deal with lingering side effects from treatment. We are not in a season of easy water in our marriage, but a season of collecting drops.

"I like it," he says. "The dress is elegant." He touches the fabric at my neck. He leans in close. "Beautiful."

I know, with three decades of assurance, he is no longer talking about dresses. Drops pool under fluorescent lights.

We stand in the downpour.

———

At the wedding, Dad escorts Mom down the grassy aisle. Our oldest son, Nate, reads a few sentences of his grandparents' peaches-and-cream love story. The guests laugh in appreciation, but mine are not the only tears, as many know of the challenges that have brought us to this day. Kevin performs the ceremony as Aleah marries her sweetheart, Todd. My husband glances my way.

I smile under the sheltering branches of desert trees.

Seven

A Hard, Forgetting Place

"Emergency Alert!" The weather app on my phone rattles in warning. I check the screen: "Dust Storm Warnings in This Area until 9:00 p.m. Avoid Travel. Check Local Media."

I go online for an updated weather report. A dust storm is traveling north from Tucson, Arizona, one hundred miles away, the second storm in a week.

I remember the year Phoenix had such a massive dust storm that meteorologists searched for another word to describe it. The experts decided on *haboob*, an Arabic word meaning "strong wind,"[1] a term usually used for describing sandstorms in the Middle East. The haboob swallowed Phoenix in a wall of dust fifty miles wide and over one mile high, traveling at speeds of fifty to sixty-five miles per hour. The next day, parking lots were covered in drifts of dirt.[2]

Summer monsoon rains have come to the high country, but not here in the Valley of the Sun. Thunder, wind, and dust—but no moisture.

I go outside to make sure the car windows are closed. The air is heavy. Thick. The horizon to the south is completely brown as clouds, trees, and houses are swallowed in a huge wave of dust. The neighbor's jacaranda tree bends in protest, purple blossoms swirling down.

Another haboob. A brown blizzard.

I hurry inside, bring in Mollie, and latch the dog door.

The storm hits right on cue as I watch from the back door. Dirt pings off the glass panels, softly at first, and then in regular staccato notes. The wind seeks entrance through every crack and crevice, whistling a siren call as it presses through tiny openings. Mollie heads to the bedroom to hide, tail between her legs.

I stand mesmerized as a section of my neighbor's roof is lifted from the back porch of his house. The shingles sail over our shared cement-block fence and twirl in a miniature dust devil in a strange, macabre dance next to our barbecue grill. After several minutes, the shingles collapse in a heap next to the swing set. With a low moan, the wind travels over our house to find its next dance partner.

The only remaining noise is the wind chime on my back porch, spinning madly in a cacophony of sound.

The storm forgot to leave water.

The desert can be a hard, forgetting place.

"We've reached the hard place in your dad's cancer," Mom tells me on the phone, repeating the words from the doctor.

Several lung tumors are no longer responding to treatment, so Dad has been taken off the clinical trial. Precise radiation is scheduled to target two tumors in his left lung. The tumors are in troublesome places—close to an airway and a major blood vessel.

Troublesome places. Hard places.

The hospital constructs a blue canoe-like container for Dad to receive treatment. The technicians cover him in a plastic-wrap material and suck the air out, encasing Dad in a body bag to keep him immobile. Only his head is free. They cannot wrap up his jokes and laughter.

A friend writes, "God is holding your dad in the palm of His hand."

My sister Renae says, "I think it's a blue cocoon, and Dad is going to go through metamorphosis and come out a new creation."

We could use life-giving changes in hard places.

As a child, I used to search for milkweed plants, the only diet for the monarch caterpillar. Then I would collect a couple of larvae, place them in a ventilated jar with a snipping of milkweed plant, and wait as each caterpillar formed a pale green chrysalis.

For about two weeks it appeared nothing was happening, but inside the chrysalis the caterpillar was changing into something completely different. In the hidden, dark place, colors changed—a caterpillar of white, yellow, and black became an orange butterfly. A creature that crawled transformed into a creation that flew. A larva that had eaten only leaves unfolded as a butterfly that drank flower nectar. A complete metamorphosis.

Maybe hard places allow God to take what is wormlike in us and give us wings to soar. Maybe in the dark, hidden places, a transformation is happening. A place where He performs personal resurrections. Where He brings peace we can't explain, but the peace is more real than the waves that rock us.

While Dad rides his blue canoe in waterless places, I am reminded of another canoe.

When I was sixteen, I went on a ten-day canoe trip in the Boundary Waters Canoe Area (BWCA) in northern Minnesota. On Saganaga Lake, the largest lake in the BWCA, where size is measured not in feet but in acres (more than seventeen thousand), we encountered a summer storm. Our aluminum canoes were tossed like toys in a bathtub, except this bathtub was 280 feet deep with waves that tumbled water over the gunwales. The wind was so strong that when we stopped paddling, our canoes traveled backward. Even paddling as hard as we could, we made little headway.

Surrounded by rolling water, the peace of the night before was forgotten. Memories of sitting around the campfire, fixing our "one pot, hot and a lot" of pasta and sharing stories of the day. Of our laughter as we set up tents by flashlight and chased out the last mosquito before climbing into sleeping bags that smelled like wood smoke. Of closing our eyes to the haunting call of the loon on flat, still waters.

Gone. All the peace of those memories. Gone.

In its place? Stark, consuming terror. A hard place.

I can relate to the disciples who screamed for help during a storm in the middle of a sea,[3] a place measured not in acres but in square miles. After feeding the five thousand, Jesus had sent them on their way across the water without him. The trip probably started easily enough, with jokes and recollections of picking up the leftovers and who had consumed the most fish and bread. Their hearts were full of seeing the miracle.

Fishermen are storytellers by trade, but I don't imagine there was any talk in the boat of the one that got away. Because it didn't get away. Hadn't they seen it with their own eyes? Two fish and a handful of loaves had fed five thousand people!

In their excitement, the disciples paid no attention to the approaching thunderclouds that blotted out the sun. Or to the descending black gloom that hung, suspended above them—waiting. Like a stick of dynamite with the fuse finally lit, the clouds exploded with rain. Drenching, soaking rain. Wind heaved the boat from side to side.

The disciples had hit a meanwhile.

"Meanwhile, the boat was far out to sea when the wind came up against them and they were battered by the waves" (Matt. 14:24 Message). Battered. For men who had made their living on this very sea, it wasn't a minor squall. It was a storm of gargantuan proportions.

The disciples were simply traveling from point A to point B, minding their own business, coming from a place of easy water, when they hit a storm.

We regularly hit meanwhiles.[4]

Meanwhile, the air conditioner is broken, the car payment is overdue, and you fear your husband wants a divorce. Meanwhile, the washing machine quit mid-cycle, your best friend isn't speaking to you, and your teenager is failing classes. Meanwhile, the car has a flat tire, the chicken soup boiled over on the stove, and your house was robbed while you ran to the grocery store.

Meanwhile . . . my dad rides in his blue canoe because he has reached a hard place with his cancer.

Meanwhile . . . I find myself in a place where circumstances have wrapped so tightly that the air has been completely sucked out and I am unable to move.

Meanwhile.

If the stories in Scripture are not only history lessons but also places we can find ourselves in the pages, where am I?

I don't have to contemplate very long before I find myself in the sentences. The disciples had spent the entire day seeing Jesus at work—preaching, healing people—and the day had climaxed with a miracle. When they found themselves in the storm, without Him, their good memories were erased. I am right there, hiding in the bottom of a boat with the disciples, cowering like my dog, Mollie, hoping the storm goes away and I am still alive at the end. After all, I am an expert at hiding. At shouting my fear: "Why did you bring me out to the desert to die?"

Storms are forgetting places. Of answered prayers. Of past provision. Of past faithfulness. Of past goodness.

Like the disciples, I have forgotten the lessons learned in the easy water of an extravagant God who provides abundantly through fish and bread, who cares for the small, and who knows everyone's name.

Are there other lessons I can learn in the story? What did Jesus do?

Right after the miracle, He sent the crowds away, He had His disciples get in a boat without Him, and He climbed a mountain to pray. Alone. After a day of hard work, of being surrounded by people on every side, Jesus made time to step away and spend time alone with His Father.

Jesus knew the discipline was vital, as essential as water.

Without the daily practice of drinking deeply from the heart of God in the times of easy water, I will be like the disciples who did not recognize Jesus coming to them in the middle of the storm, who did not know their own dear friend.

"When my prayer life suffers, my ability to trust God during the storms of life also suffers. If I wait until I think I have time, I will never slip off to the quiet places. Thus, when the storms arrive, I look out through the turbulence and see only the ghost of God," Macrina Wiederkehr writes.[5]

"I look out through the turbulence and see only the ghost of God." The disciples thought Jesus was a ghost out there in the storm. A ghost. Something dead from the past. A long ago memory. Nobody with power or answers to help them.

In the middle of a storm, a memory, a ghost of a relationship, won't help me. The disciples found this to be true. In the middle of their meanwhile, in their terror, they cried out for help from a friend, only to discover He was God.

I need a living, breathing encounter. I need a relationship that is vibrant and real. I need "a desperate dependence on the present voice of God."[6] I need a metamorphosis for my cowering heart. Only then will I hear His voice coming from the middle of the storm. "Take courage, it is I; do not be afraid" (Matt. 14:27).

I hear the words. I want to believe them. I battle with the waves of fear and doubt as my dad rides his blue canoe in the hard reality of cancer. I survey the brewing storm.

Where is Jesus, my dear friend?

Eight

Difficult Beauty

Spring skipped the desert this year.

You wouldn't know it by the temperature. While the rest of the country struggles to dig out of the biggest freeze of the century, we in Arizona have logged day after day of temperate weather. The sweaters have been packed away and . . . what is a snow blower anyway?

Spring skipped the desert this year.

You wouldn't know it by the landscaped grass and drip-lined flowers. Lawn mowers are being tuned. Pink oleander and fuchsia bougainvillea bushes are in full bloom. Citrus trees have lost their white flowers to be replaced by minuscule green orbs hidden in thorny branches.

Spring skipped the desert this year.

Outside the city, away from irrigated properties, the ground did not receive adequate rain. Poppy seeds, without the necessary moisture, tucked in tight for another twelve months, holding the vow to bloom again. I miss the delicate orange beauty dotting the continuous brown canvas.

The sturdier brittlebush and desert daisy managed on the limited rain, yet already, their yellow petals have come and gone.

Under the beating rays of the relentless sun, without the relief of rain, the hard-worn paths of the desert have grayed down, subdued into endless tans and browns, adding a fierceness to a land already known for its struggle to exist. The landscape is raw, unfinished.

No splashes of purple. No breaks of orange. No breath of pink.

Only muted brown everywhere. The gauntness of the half-starved dirt is broken occasionally by jutting boulders and bare mountains.

Color can be found in only one place.

The sky. The dawn begins deep blue, nearly purple, as the stars go to bed for another day. Near sunrise the sky boldens to intense yellow and orange. For most of the day, the sky is blue.

But oh, what an intense, incredible blue!

With no other color in the artist's palette, the blue of the desert sky is breathtaking. Usually unbroken by any clouds, the desert blue is deep and endless, stretching unlimited above.

You can dive into the blueness.

People generally describe the desert as a place to be avoided. Survived. The barrenness is a place of fear. Mistrust. Pain. Some would even call the desert *godforsaken*. At best, travelers are only passing through, searching for an escape, a homecoming to a place of easy water.

I have been that desert wanderer. I have only seen the desolation, without the beauty. I have languished under one hundred–degree skies. I have longed for the day we would move and plant our roots elsewhere.

"To stand before both the difficult and the beautiful with an open heart will take some practice,"[1] Macrina Wiederkehr writes in *Seven Sacred Pauses*. In such standing, I am still an amateur.

On a visit to see my parents, Mom and Dad take me to view several condos and apartments in town as they contemplate selling their country acreage. Mom creates a spreadsheet of what the different places will cost and how much income would be available if one or both of them are still living.

"Could you be happy here without me?" Mom asks Dad as they tour a fourth prospective apartment. They stand near a large bay window overlooking the lake in town.

"I can't imagine being happy anywhere without you," Dad says.

"Well, where do you want to live?" Mom asks, trying to tie Dad to a decision.

"Heaven."

Sometimes as an eavesdropper on my parents' love story, I discover the difficult and the beautiful are one and the same. As I stand witness to their final chapter, in all its tenderness and challenges, I struggle to keep my heart open. I want many more years of practice.

For the first time in my life I understand the meaning of bittersweet. It shares the shade with difficult beauty.

As a child, our younger daughter, Katelyn, disliked hiking and would do anything in her power to avoid the activity. A trip to the Havasu Canyon when she was seven was no exception, but we hoped the thirty other backpackers in the group, many who were also children, would distract her. My husband had the role of sweeper, going last in the group to make sure nobody was left behind. Wanting to put miles into energetic little legs, I set out, without him, on the ten-mile hike with the children.

The first few miles were fun as the kids skipped down the trail, running ahead to hide behind rocks and jumping out to scare one another. We left behind the switchbacks, dropping two thousand feet of elevation in one mile, to where the path flattened. We hiked in the dry wash, bordered by red sandstone cliffs in the narrow canyon. The monotony of the miles took its toll. Our older two, both teens, jogged ahead to hike with friends. I found myself carrying Zach, age five, while his sister wanted to take a break every ten steps.

Katelyn finally stopped altogether and sprawled flat on the dusty trail.

"Just leave me here," she begged.

No amount of pleading, threatening, or bargaining could get her to budge. I didn't know what to do.

But then Kevin appeared behind us. He quickly assessed the situation. He put Zach on his shoulders and reached his hand toward his daughter.

She looked up.

Into the face of her father.

"Let's go," he said. "You can get whatever you want to drink at the village store."

Katelyn dusted herself off, took his hand, and off we ventured down the trail toward three days of adventure—splashing in waterfalls, camping, swimming, descending cliff faces, and making memories. But first, we stopped at the store as promised. Katelyn chose grape soda.

Throughout the years, our family has teased her about that day, but now, years later, I understand the heart of my daughter.

I am in a season of more than I can handle. I can't imagine taking one more step, let alone walking for miles and miles into another day. I have days when the only thing I want is to lie down in the middle of my life and say, "Just leave me here." Days when I don't know what to do or where to turn. Exhausting, mind-numbing, worn-out, tiring, dust-eating, discouraging days.

People like to say, "God won't give you more than you can handle." The words are spoken after another health crisis hits and everyone—my friends, my family, my church community, my sixth cousin five times removed—is trying to help me cope with a new reality. The phrase is meant to be reassuring, but I've decided it is a lie.

It's blatantly untrue, because if I never had more than I could handle, when would I ever need God?

Every day in this season of more than I can handle, I run out of me. I juggle life as a mom, friend, wife, daughter, and woman with various jobs and responsibilities. I am stretched too thin. The challenge remains: Will I run to God? He can handle whatever is more than I can handle. In fact, He even handles what I think I am capable of handling, only to discover I am not.

"The LORD is like a strong tower; those who do right can run to him for safety" (Prov. 18:10 NCV). Running is not enough. I need to race toward Jesus in a flat-out sprint.

———

"What are you currently reading?" the lady asks me at the church potluck, while I balance a plate of baked beans, chicken salad, and watermelon.

"A book on the desert," I say. "Not a spiritual book, but written by a naturalist."

She nods in understanding. "The natural world and spiritual world are often connected."

I step closer, encouraged by the interest in her voice. "I have always thought the desert is something to escape," I confess. "Now I wonder if the desert has beauty that can only be discovered here. Difficult beauty."

"I have lived most of my life in the desert. Everyone else saw only brown. I always found it beautiful."

My heart contemplates the words of this woman who has lived in northern Africa, away from family and all that is familiar, who has told other people about Jesus in a barren place. I wonder what beauty she has found there.

"In the book," I say, "the author says that all the parts of the desert—the canyons, the washes, and the ravines—point to where water has flowed. The boulders, the mountains, and the arroyos serve as conduits when there is water."[2]

She smiles. "I will have to think about that all week."

I take a mouthful of watermelon. Swallow down the sweetness. I know I need to meditate on the words. Am I a conduit of water in the desert? What is flowing out of me? Through me?

Standing next to platters of fried chicken and potato salad, I find a heart connection with a fellow desert sojourner who has searched for water and beauty in difficult places. "I believe some lessons from God can only be discovered here," I say. The words come out tentatively, as if they have traveled a long journey and have only now been released to the light of day.

Her eyes hold the knowledge of one who knows. "'I will win her back once again,'" she quotes. "'I will lead her into the desert and speak tenderly to her there.'"[3] She clears her throat. "God woos us in the desert."

I want to continue the conversation, but we are separated by someone needing a cup of lemonade. My heart ponders her words. I have felt the wooing. My heart has resisted as I have lain in desert dust, viewing only the difficult and not the beauty. *Just leave me here!*

What does the Wooer of my soul want to teach me in the desert? Can I open my heart to hear His tender words? Is it possible this desert is a place of incredible beauty?

Naturalist Craig Childs is frequently told the desert is a horrible place. He admits there is truth to that statement, but "within the horror, in time spent, a person learns the languages and voice. The dialogue is unending."[4] Too often I am guilty of hearing a monologue—my own—as I stumble to find my way. Oh, how I want to hear the unending voice of He who loves me.

———

I am not the only one who has been taken on a desert journey. Jesus was led out to the desert by the Spirit of God immediately after His baptism in the Jordan River by His cousin John.[5] When Jesus stepped out from the water, His skin dripping wet, leaving dampness in the dirt, He heard His Father speak of His pleasure in Jesus as His much-loved Son.

Jesus left a place of easy water, a place of hearing the voice of God. And where did He then find Himself?

Before the imprints from His feet could dry, Jesus was led into the desert. No food for forty days and nights. The Evil Whisperer tempted with his words of mistrust. Rather than the voice of His Father, Jesus heard the voice of Satan, who issued a dare that involved turning stones into bread. "If you are the Son of God," the tempter taunted.

This is the same challenge I face in desert places. Whose voice will I listen to? Will I listen to the One who woos me and takes pleasure in me, or will I hear the voice of the Evil Whisperer who tempts me to distrust God's goodness and care? Or do I, instead, grab on to my own strength and take care of myself?

Jesus remembered the words of His Father. "Man shall not live on bread alone, but on every word that comes from the mouth of God" (Matt. 4:4 NIV).

Whose voice do I hear? Will I cling to desert dust, clutching stones, hoping they will become bread? Will I see only the difficult? The impossible?

I sense His coming. I simply need to look up. His hand extends to me where I have flung myself in desert dust, crying, "Just leave me here!"

I hear the wooing, the tender words. I stretch out my fingers.

I can't imagine being happy anywhere without you.

I wonder if He knows the best place to find grape soda.

Nine

A Stack of Gratitude Stones

A white-winged dove greets the dawn underneath the light of a banana moon. Kevin and I cross a dry desert wash, the stones, like the vegetation, gray and uninviting. We head east, past a thin blanket strung from an ironwood tree, the remnant of an abandoned childhood fort. Brittlebush, creosote, and cactus dot the sparse landscape. Our surroundings shift to brown as we head down the trail. We hike straight into the new morning.

The plan is to take the Pyramid Trail until it joins the National and Busera Trails, a hike in the Gila Range at South Mountain Preserve in Phoenix. We cross the dry arroyo three times before reaching the switchbacks. The first shaft of light hits the peaks before melting down like butter into the valleys. The day begins without fanfare. No oranges. No golds. Only the palest of yellow.

Three miles in and I stop, exhausted. My lungs burn. My breath comes heavy. The weight of worry presses against my shoulders as I climb, step after weary step. I have not hiked long enough to be tired, but my body is spent. Countless sleepless nights have caught up with me.

Yesterday, Mom sent an email with the news her white blood cell count was low, putting her at risk for infection. Her body is not recovering fast enough in between chemo treatments. Dad's tumors have grown two millimeters. Twenty percent. Melanoma is figuring out a way to grow around the meds. The doctor wants to run more tests. I took out a ruler to remind myself how tiny two millimeters is.

"It's only two millimeters," I tell myself as I trudge on. How can something so minuscule stir so much emotion? So much fear? Cancer has taken a magnifying glass to my emotions. An amplifier. Fear. Anger. Hope. Helplessness. Courage. Despair. I have experienced them all.

Kevin pulls farther and farther ahead as I continue to struggle up the incline. Mollie keeps pace with him, but then dashes back to check on me, unsure what to do. She does this several times as my husband continues to climb, oblivious, up the mountain.

Anger burns within me. Grief wears a mask and comes out to find fault. That Kevin is familiar with my habit of lagging behind to take photos, and then catching up, does nothing to appease me. Today I want him to be a mind reader, to know I need to go slower, to know I need rest.

To know I need . . . him.

Finally fed up, I stop on a rock outcropping. I take off my pack and collapse, not caring that Kevin is hiking on without me or that he won't know I stopped. I eat an apple and a package of fruit snacks. Fifteen minutes go by.

The jingle of Mollie's dog tags alerts me to their return.

"Are you all right?" Kevin asks, his forehead creased with worry.

"Just tired." I don't want to get into it.

"There's a shortcut ahead."

I sigh and stumble to my feet. I hitch my backpack over my shoulders and head up the trail. I know it is my best option for getting back to the car, but I don't like it. Usually our hikes are filled with chatter.

Not today. The silence is oppressive.

I want words. He doesn't have any.

We pass a toppled barrel cactus on the side of the trail. The roots lie exposed, the four-foot cactus split in two. The pieces lay dried and brittle on the desert floor. Only the fishhook spines remain on the dead shell.

I stop to take photos, from several angles, while Kevin pours Mollie a drink of water in her collapsible water dish. The cactus strikes a chord with me. Burned out. Toppled. Spines snag as anger curls and hooks.

Words come slowly as we continue on the trail. I stumble over my words, expressing my fear and anxiety about my parents. About the future. About the crushing weight of the unknown. And the known. Sentences spill faster as I seek to unhook what has pricked deep into my soul. My husband slows his pace to match mine as we hike several miles.

The words finally dwindle to an end. A hummingbird whirs past me in search of nectar, his speeding wings the only sound besides our crunching footsteps. I focus on Kevin, expecting a response.

"You should say something," I say, hoping a nudge will prompt conversation.

He blows his air out in a compressed sigh. "What do you want me to say?"

Anger tries to rehook. "Say that it's going to be okay." I speak the words in exasperation, knowing they are lame, but I have no better solutions.

His hazel eyes fill with light. "I can do that." He grins. "It's going to be okay."

"That's not what I meant."

"It's going to be okay," he repeats.

I want to glare, but something inside me loosens and I smile instead, because isn't this the man who has already lost two parents to cancer? Didn't he help care for his mother in her last few weeks of life? Isn't he living proof that one day I will breathe again? That there is a life beyond impending loss?

"There it is," he says.

"There what is?" I ask, jostled from my ponderings.

"The shortcut," he says, pointing to a cairn on the downside of the trail. I scrutinize the short stack of rocks. I see no well-worn path beyond, only a slight indention in the surrounding mountainside. Few feet have traveled here.

"Are you sure?" I ask.

Kevin unfolds a topographical map, the squiggly lines indicating the rise and fall of elevations. He is old school and does not like GPS. He traces the trail with his finger, stopping on the spot corresponding to where we now stand. He nods.

Sometimes cairns are in predictable spots, but this cairn has been placed by travelers who have marked a way that is not obvious.

We take the shortcut and return home. For several days, whenever Kevin catches my eye, he grins. "It's going to be okay," he says. He kisses my neck when I am doing dishes and whispers it quietly in my ear. He says it before he heads off to work in the morning. He glances up from the computer and says it. "It's going to be okay."

Something inside unhooks and uncurls. It's as if Kevin gathers stones and stacks them on top of each other, one by one with each repetition of the phrase, marking the way that is not obvious through this trail of grief.

My heart hears the words—"it's going to be okay"—the answer to an unspoken question, a question I have been too afraid to ask.

We are going to be okay.

———

Dad purchases a white convertible. A "bucket list car," he calls it. "Are you coming home to Minnesota because you think I'm going to die?" Dad asks me on the phone when I call.

"No," I reply, "I'm coming to ride in your car."

And ride we do.

We ride to town for groceries. I drive to meet a friend for coffee. We take photos of the grandkids as they each take a turn in the driver's seat. And one night—just because—we pile into the car and cruise to town to get ice cream.

Afterward, we take the long way home, meandering our way past a church, a dusk-shadowed lake, and miles and miles of cornfields. The wind flings my hair in all directions. The strands escape any attempt of containment. Mom offers me a headband, but I decide to let it fly.

Uncontrolled. Uncontained. Unrestrained.

In a white convertible, on a wind-whipped night, during a desert journey that began with the phone call saying it was cancer, joy finds me. Unexpected joy.

With the top down, I discover the reason for keeping a gratitude journal, a rationale for recording the daily thanks, at least three reasons each day. I began the discipline after Dad's diagnosis. It is not a kindergarten exercise of writing "I'm thankful for the color purple" or "I'm thankful for spaghetti."

It is deeper than that. Thankfulness is not given in a void. Thankfulness is given to Someone. To God. It is a yielding, a bending, a trusting He is in control. The giving of thanks is the result of a submitted life.

In Hebrews, it says, "At present we do not yet see all things under his control."[1] On this earth we still deal with illness. Wars and evil. Pain. Loss. Days I pray for healing and nights I scream, "Cancer stinks, and it can't have my dad! Or my mom!"

Wind-whipped times.

Scripture continues, "But we do see Jesus."[2] I am not left alone in the darkness. My eyes need to be opened to see Him. I believe this seeing, this eye-opening even in the dark, begins with a heart of gratitude, the daily giving of thanks. Right here. Right now.

As I gather rocks and stack them, one by one, I hear the whisper "It's going to be okay." I give thanks, on good days and bad, and build a cairn to mark the way. On days the path is not clear, when

I travel where few feet have gone, I gather another stone. Fellow sojourners who walk this trail choose gratitude and goodness in the midst of life's difficulties as they chart a new way through the desert.

Perhaps this is also why Jesus had his disciples gather crumbs—not only to remember the miracle, but with each bending of their knees, the disciples were training their hearts to be present to the reality of now, to see a God who is I AM and the giver of all good gifts. "'God is good' is not some trite quip for the good days but a radical defiant cry for the terrible days . . . a saving lifeline when all's hard,"[3] author Ann Voskamp writes.

Thankfulness is a topographical map for the rise and fall on desert journeys. When all is difficult, gratitude is the cairn that marks the way.

On the day I was first diagnosed, I wrote in my journal. With shaking fingers, I penned,

> God is good.
> This is a settled fact in my heart.
> It's not cross-my-fingers-and-hope-it's-true wishful thinking.
> It's not a someday-I'll-see-it-but-not-until-I-die mournful statement.
> It's not religious words murmured as a talisman against evil.
> It's a fact.
> Settled.
> Established.
> Fixed in my heart.
> God is good.
> And today?
> It is enough.

On that first day of my diagnosis, I mentally collected a stone and put it in my pocket. The edges are worn smooth now from the handling. When my parents were diagnosed, I pulled out the stone. I discovered it is one thing to trust your own life to the hand of God; it is a completely different matter to trust Him with those you love.

So I pull out the stone, not to throw in anger or to slay a giant. I place the stone at the base of a new cairn. To mark the way. As I do, I hear the voice of Jesus. In His words I hear the answer to the question I have been afraid to ask. The soft words uncurl and unhook something inside me.

"We are going to be okay."

Ten

Laughter and Faith
Hold Hands

My mother is an exceptional gardener. Four extensive flower beds of perennials—lilies, peonies, tulips—color their property. Two wooden tubs of pink petunias spill out a welcome at the main entrance. "Bubblegum petunias," Mom says, and she would know, because she keeps a notebook of all the flowers, their names, and a record of when and where they were planted. Shopping for her Mother's Day gift is easy—every year, the four of us siblings pitch in for a gift certificate to the local nursery.

I did not inherit my mom's green thumb. The standing joke around our family is that plants come here for hospice care. I figure I have time to keep the plants alive or my children, and so far my children are winning.

The one plant that has survived all my attempts to kill it has been the cat's claw vine in the backyard. The vine, known for its drought tolerance, weaves its way up the slatted ramada, completely shading the back porch. Each spring, masses of trumpet-shaped yellow flowers cascade down. The vines have not yet bloomed when my parents come for another visit.

My dad stands under the arching cat's claw vine on a perfect January desert night. He positions his handwritten note so he can catch the glow from the strands of twinkling lights entwined in the branches. He has traveled sixteen hundred miles to give our youngest a gift at his eighteenth birthday party—the passing of a spiritual blessing from an older generation to a younger one.

For months we talked about the possibility of my parents coming.

"We can connect you to Skype for the party," I told my mom, "or call you on the phone."

"We will come if we are up to it," Mom said. I knew her words were true, but I also knew how much "it" we were talking about, so I tried not to get my hopes up.

When Dad stands before the party guests, I wonder what words of wisdom and blessing he will share with our son Zach. What do you travel sixteen hundred miles to say? Do you talk about integrity? Honor? Courage? Finding a job you love? The importance of hard work? Of honesty?

Dad talks about none of these things.

Dad talks about laughter. The power of joy. Of not focusing on cancer, but on discovering reasons to smile every day.

I watch this man who has loved me for more than fifty years speak wisdom to my son. I know I am hearing the heartbeat of his life, for this is a man who jokes with his oncologist and gets the nurses laughing. When my husband asked him for my hand in marriage three decades ago, Dad's only stipulation was "Make my daughter happy."

He clears his throat and readjusts his page to the light. Does he choke back emotion or the damage in his lungs from melanoma? I'm not sure.

A never-ending cough has gripped his body and is wearing him down. Earlier in the week he had to pause to catch his breath when he climbed the one flight of steps to our daughter's apartment. He sleeps in a chair to reduce the coughing and is on his fourth super-plus-giant-size bag of cough drops.

"'A joyful heart is good medicine,'" Dad reads, "'but a broken spirit dries up the bones.'"[1] He turns to Zach. "Pursue laughter," he says. "Find reasons for joy."

Then he sits down. But not without telling a one-liner that makes the guests laugh.

My mother stands to share her blessing, her head wrapped fashionably in a turquoise scarf.

I remember, months ago, when she emailed us photos of her bald head, shaved the same day Zach was chosen as homecoming king. While our son's friends cheered and applauded on the football field, Mom's crown fell in ringlets on the linoleum. I thought, *This is a snapshot of my crazy life, where I have a high school son receiving accolades and a mom starting chemo—and they both carry crowns. One worn. One shorn.*

Isn't this everyone's life, learning to live with the wild up and down of it all? We each have moments when we stand straight, tall, and proud, confident in our accomplishments and the appreciation of others; when we smile in the mirror, tilt the crown jauntily on our head, and shout, "I'm on top of the world!"

But then there are the days when our crowns fall in pieces at our feet, leaving us skin-bare, stripped down, and hesitant at the words we hear whispered in our heart's reflections. And isn't one of life's toughest lessons learning that who you really are is never about what is on your head?

Mom stands to address the party guests, with her turquoise scarf and her missing eyebrows drawn in place. On her feet are slippers, because her feet are too swollen to put on shoes, and in her hand is a Kleenex to wipe her constantly dripping nose, a side effect of losing her nose hairs to chemo.

What do you travel sixteen hundred miles to say? What grips your heart so you schedule your chemo the morning of your flight and then get on a plane to come speak words over your grandson?

Do you talk about love? Of sacrifice? Of finding the perfect life mate?

Mom talks about none of these things.

She unfolds a paper and speaks words found in Psalm 139. She tells our son he is fearfully and wonderfully made by God, that his heavenly Father has a plan and purpose for his life only He can fulfill. He is not an accident and God has incredible days written in His book, future chapters and destinies to walk out.

I listen to this woman who is several more chapters into her life story than my son. I know I am hearing the heartbeat of her life—of generations who have followed God and who have chosen faith in difficult times; a woman who now leaves a heritage to her children's children.

"All this is God's plan," Mom says to our son. "We don't know everything about who you are going to be or what you are going to do, but you are loved. You are a blessing to your family and you are a life-giver in the world."

She returns to Dad's side. They intertwine fingers.

Laughter and faith hold hands as they sit under the cat's claw vine in the backyard, a vine that has withstood the heat and drought of many summers. For fifty-five years of marriage, love has triumphed over adversity, and when given the opportunity, our son's grandparents travel sixteen hundred miles to speak this legacy of blessing to him.

———

"DONE" the subject line reads on Mom's latest email after they return to Minnesota. I click to read it:

Today marked the completion of my five months of chemo. The scans indicate the cancer is gone. We celebrated with bell ringing, chocolates, listening to the singing card sent by all of you, and beautiful flowers. Thank you family for everything you have done in the past months—your prayers, your cards and your gifts, your words of compassion, your phone calls, and your hugs. I shed a few tears as I thanked the nursing staff for their care these last months.

We have turned a new page in our lives. The Lord is my light and my salvation. . . . . The Lord is the strength of my life, of whom (or what) should I be afraid.

I try to continue reading the rest of the email, of chatty news about their lives, but I have to stop. Joy has taken over my eyes. The emotion travels over the internet and trickles down my cheeks. When I try to read the email to my family, joy escapes again and clogs my throat. How do you put into words what you hoped was true but were afraid to believe because you didn't want to be disappointed?

It's a spring of joy type of day.

When my husband and I lived in the Boundary Waters in Minnesota, we lived near Hungry Jack Springs, a natural spring that bubbles out of an area covered in ferns and wildflowers. Hanging from a low branch next to the spring was a metal cup you could use to get a drink, but I preferred to dip my hands into the icy coldness, bringing the refreshing water to my lips and drinking deeply.

The water tasted like a hundred snowfalls.

All day, after reading Mom's email, a spring of joy bubbles inside me, like a shaken can of soda waiting to explode sticky sweetness all around. I pay no attention to my inner librarian who says, "Shhh! Quiet down!"

Springs of joy cannot be contained.

A sparrow builds a nest under the eaves in the branches of the cat's claw vine. She lays three speckled eggs.

Six weeks go by. Only forty-two days under desert sun.

Mom's latest scans aren't good. The cancer is back. Or was never gone. Dad's cancer moves to his brain. Doctors throw together words like *palliative* and *hospice* and *Dad* in the same sentence.

I get off the phone with Mom. I step outside onto the back porch and glare at the sun shining in a cloudless sky. A stormy day would better fit my mood, as I stand, unmoving. Wasn't it only a few weeks ago when my dad told jokes and spoke a blessing on this same porch?

I collapse on the cement step, my head between my knees. It's as if the air is too thin to breathe. There is no bubbly soda today. The lid is off and I am flat. I replay the conversation over and over in my mind.

Cancer returned. Brain tumors. Hospice. No amount of replaying changes the tune.

Several minutes pass before a silvery shrill pierces my numb brain. The mama sparrow is not happy with my proximity to her nest.

I stumble to a standing position, thankful for something to do. Anything. Anything to drown out the words. I check the nest under the bright trumpet flowers. Empty.

Four days ago, on a Sunday, the three baby birds explored the edge of the nest, peeping loudly as they ventured out from the hollowed safety. Monday, I saw one on the block wall when I walked into the alley, his baby feathers sticking out from his head like a bad hair day. His sibling bobbed frantically in a corner of the woodpile. I grabbed Mollie, the bird-chasing dog, by the collar and dragged her inside. The third fledgling had already flown away.

On Tuesday, we rescued woodpile birdie from the backyard garbage can. Twice. We untangled him from the cat's claw vine, where he fled in terror. We placed him back on the woodpile in hopes he would practice his flying lessons. Mollie was quarantined to the house.

So now I check the yard. The woodpile. The garbage can. I cannot find him. The baby sparrow has taken to the skies.

I remember Dad singing in church when I was a girl. He sang a song about sparrows and God watching over them. He loved the song because his father—my grandfather—a crusty old dairy farmer, sang the hymn while milking the cows.

Grandpa always had one or two cows he liked to milk by hand. He would position the milk stool, grab a teat in each hand, and—swish, swish, swish—the milk would squirt into the bucket with a practiced cadence. The barn cats would come running from the haymow and other dark corners of the barn and encircle my grandfather's feet.

Grandpa would tilt a teat and squirt a stream of warm milk into each waiting cat's mouth. While he milked he sang a song about God watching over the birds. My grandfather sang the song. My dad learned the song by the repetition of his father's words.

On my back porch I think of baby fledglings and am reminded that God, who doesn't forget the birds, has not forgotten us. Sometimes on hard days—no, correction, especially on hard days—God encounters us with His love.

The enormity of the words I have just heard spoken on the phone are suddenly eclipsed with the weightedness of *presence*. The comforting wordlessness of Jesus encounters me under the sparrow's nest. He comes in a way that is personal and intimate, that speaks of love and life to *me*. Who else would know the story of my father and grandfather? The significance of the sparrows?

I sit surrounded in a love-encountering moment.

Here under the cat's claw vine, God comes with a personal love message. He comes with baby birds.

"Are not five sparrows sold for two pennies? Yet not one of them is forgotten by God. Indeed, the very hairs of your head are all numbered. Don't be afraid; you are worth more than many sparrows" (Luke 12:6–7 NIV).

You are worth more than many sparrows.

If the value of something can be found in what someone is willing to pay for it, then I am overwhelmed by this numbers-loving God who does not forget five-for-two-pennies sparrows, yet sent His Son to pay with His life—for me. Even on this most miserable day, I hear the invitation to step off the edge of all that is known and believe in a God who loves, a God who loves, a God who loves.

Don't be afraid.

Even here. Even now.

Can I spread my fingers wide and let go of one more level of control? Can I trust myself and my dad to what I cannot yet see? Can I leave the hallowed safety?

Dad stands on the edge.

Eleven

Remember the Sound of Rain

The sound of thunder wakes me. The digital numbers in the dark room glow 3:58. I turn to go back to sleep, but with the thunder, I hear another sound.

Could that be rain?

The thought draws me out of my pillowed comfort to investigate. The months have been dry. A slight scattering of rain fell a few weeks ago, but the ground has received no moisture since then. Dry as dust. So much dust. The weather has seduced us with storm clouds, but we have had only dry thunderstorms. Long tails have streamed from high clouds with the promise of rain, but the moisture evaporated before it hit the ground due to the low humidity and high temperatures.

We are in the waiting, when it can be difficult to hold on to promises. To hold on to hope. Every day clouds mushroom the skies, but we are left standing in the dust.

To the non-desert dweller, the excitement found in the arrival of rain may seem a strange phenomenon. We have abandoned puzzled dinner guests at the table in order to stand in the front yard, our faces lifted skyward for the falling.

Our youngest was seven months old before he experienced his first rainstorm. It was August and we had ridden the chairlift at Snowbowl up the western slope of Humphreys Peak, the tallest peak in Arizona (12,633 feet). We hiked part of the summit trail, the kids searching for the distinct orange-red bark of the ponderosa pine so they could sniff the vanilla scent found in the trunk. The trees thinned as we climbed in elevation, but before we made the alpine tundra, we glanced at the sky—dreary and threatening. A storm was brewing.

Kevin took the boys and I had the girls with me as we get on the chairlift for the twenty-five-minute descent. The wind picked up as we soared above the forest, the pines exhaling in the moist pregnant air. Halfway down, the thunderstorm hit, wild and furious, pelting us from all sides. We scrambled to put on raincoats on our narrow, swinging perches.

And then . . . the power shut down.

We hung suspended in space on the chairlift with no place to hide. The rain came at us sideways, drenching us in seconds.

And then . . . the lightning.

Around us, lightning zigzagged while we sat with front-row seats to nature's display of raw power. I watched petrified, fully aware we were now the highest landmark in an electrically charged landscape.

Lightning blazed, thunder exploded, the wind ranted, and, according to Kevin, our young son laughed. Zach peered out from the protection of his dad's raincoat and stretched his fingers to touch the falling water. Soon that wasn't enough. He opened his mouth to catch the rain. He wasn't content to merely touch the water; he wanted to totally experience it.

After that incident (yes, we did get down safely and the lodge gave us free hot cocoa), Zach could not get enough of rain. Whenever he saw a puddle, he did not simply splash his feet with toddler exuberance. Instead, he would lie down, face flat to the concrete, connecting as much skin as possible to the water, as if his pores needed to remember the feel of rain. The smell. The essence.

These memories draw me now from my bed. The promise of rain.

I open the front door to the blackness. A welcome sound blankets me. Gentle. Cleansing. Rain.

Still in my jammies, I sit outside on the bench under the eaves and watch the water fall. The lightning parade. Drops hiss as they bounce off the steaming asphalt. The rain hits the sidewalk and splashes my bare feet. For forty minutes I sit and soak up the sound as the rain falls. The soothing cadence drips into the dry cracks of my soul, weaving its way into the hard places.

The shower descends on plant carcasses. Thirsty ground. Endless concrete heat.

And one tired heart.

———

In John 11, Jesus receives word His friend Lazarus is sick. Jesus doesn't leave right away but purposely delays. Author Ken Gire writes, "Jesus doesn't rush to his bedside. Not because he is too busy. Or because he doesn't care. But because the Father is orchestrating an incredible moment and needs time to set the stage. And since a corpse must be center stage before this drama can begin, Jesus must wait until Lazarus dies before He can make His entrance."[1]

Unfortunately, Lazarus's sisters, Mary and Martha, can't see behind the curtain. They can't see the director's notes. The sisters see only the gathering darkness. "They sit at home, despondent, as in an empty theater, their tearful prayers returning to them like hollow echoes off indifferent walls."[2]

The Evil Whisperer repeats his memorized lies, the words of doubt in a God who loves, either questioning His power or His compassion. The Evil Whisperer once spoke the phrases in the Garden of Eden and then again in a wilderness where stones masqueraded as loaves of bread. The words vary, but the message is always the same: *Did God really say He loved you? Who are you kidding? If Jesus is God, why doesn't He come heal your brother? Your father? Your friend? He cares about other people, but where is He now?* The mental torment escalates. We all have our questions.

When Jesus and the disciples finally arrive, they discover Lazarus has been dead four days. Martha goes out to meet Jesus first. She greets Him with these words: "Lord, if You had been here, my brother would not have died" (John 11:21). After a brief discussion, Martha goes to get her sister. Mary comes out, sees Jesus, and falls at His feet. "Lord, if You had been here, my brother would not have died" (John 11:32).

Two sisters. Same words. The Bible doesn't say how Martha made her comment to Christ, so this is speculation, but I believe since her posture is not mentioned and Mary's is mentioned, that Martha spoke face-to-face with Jesus. I know my own disillusionment in circumstances of pain and grief. And I know how I have responded. "Lord, if You had been here . . ." I have done my own speaking in God's face in regard to cancer.

Cancer has turned me into a hater. I hate cancer. Cancer steals, kills, and destroys. There is nothing romantic about cancer, even when we tie it up in different colored ribbons. Pink for breast cancer. Black for melanoma. Teal for ovarian. Before cancer, I associated ribbons with gift giving.

Some find comfort in viewing cancer as a gift from God. I understand the struggle to put words and meaning to the incomprehensible, but I struggle with this image of cancer. When someone tells me they have cancer, I don't say, "Oh, lucky you, you got a present!" I want to slap something. And point them to customer service to return this "gift."

Cancer makes me angry.

I join Martha on a dusty road, and I stare directly into His face and wonder why He wasn't there. Because if He had been there—been here—Dad and Mom wouldn't be dying before my eyes. I want to draw a line in the sand at the unfairness of it all and scream, "No more!"

The clouds build, the darkness descends, and I question God's love. Oswald Chambers writes, "Unless we can look the darkest, blackest fact full in the face without damaging God's character, we do not yet know him."[3]

I stand shoulder to shoulder with Martha.

How does Jesus respond to Martha? Does He frown, scold her for her words? Put her in her place?

Jesus does none of that. Jesus speaks hope. He says, "Your brother will rise again" (John 11:23).

Jesus goes on to say He is the resurrection; that everyone who believes in Him will never die. First hope. Then life. Jesus speaks words of life. He is not afraid of her questions.

And He is not afraid of my questions. Of my doubts. "Never doubt that there are two kinds of doubt," Ann Voskamp writes, "one that fully lives into the questions and one that uses the questions as weapons against fully living."[4]

Holocaust survivor Elie Wiesel said, "My questioning of God goes on. But even from the beginning I believed in questioning God from inside faith, not from outside faith. It is because I believe that I am all the time questioning."[5]

Inside faith, I want to fully live in my questions.

What about Mary? How does she respond? "Lord, if You had been here, my brother would not have died" (John 11:32). Mary responds with the same words, but bent low, prostrate in the dust, her grief overcoming her.

I have lain in the dust with Mary, utterly broken. I have come to Jesus, the only one who can heal what is shattered. I understand Mary, because I have wept my own words at His feet, "Jesus, please don't let cancer take my mom and dad."

I am Martha. I am Mary. I stand and speak questions in the face of Jesus and in the next breath speak words of belief and truth.

And I am so overcome with grief all I can do is fall at His feet and weep the agony of my impending loss.

But I take heart. The two sisters—one who says the words to Jesus's face and one who says the words to His feet—move the heart of Christ and He weeps.

I don't know what is more wondrous: Jesus who is able to raise the dead or Jesus who cries as God. Both are needed.

Without both the power and the compassion, we are lost. It's easy for me to imagine a God who is powerful. Who tosses around lightning bolts and roars with thunder. Who speaks a single word and it is done. But a God who cries?

In that cry, I hear, "It was not supposed to be like this. Your hearts were not fashioned for grief. They were created for relationship. For love. For foreverness. For unbrokenness. You were not created to stand at the edge of a grave."

In that cry is our hope. Our salvation. Our gift. Not cancer. Jesus.

The cry brought God to a manger, to a tomb of a dear friend, and eventually to a cross. Jesus didn't walk away. He could have walked away from Martha. From Mary. He could have walked away from me. If He had turned His back, there would be no hope. But He didn't. He is still moved with compassion.

But Jesus didn't stop with tears.

For this is God, who is not only compassionate but also powerful—who once interrupted a funeral procession to raise a widow's son right out of his coffin, who breathed with his Father and the Spirit into the barren wombs of Sarah and Elizabeth and Hannah. Who escorted the mourners outside the home of Jairus and then held the hand of Jairus's daughter and said, "Child arise," and restored the girl to her amazed parents. This is the God who came to this earth in human form, for the determined purpose of overcoming death, which held humankind in its grip and made us captive.

So the slight complication of a dead body doesn't sway Jesus now. Jesus walks to the entrance of a four-day-old sealed tomb with the smell of death in the air. Death of a dream. Death of hope. Death of a future. Death of a body. He stands where compassion and power unite and speaks resurrection life, and suddenly we have a dead man walking.

In the hands of God, in the hands of Jesus, death is only the prelude to resurrection,[6] if not now, then in eternity.

Hebrews 6:19–20 says, "This hope we have as an anchor of the soul, a hope both sure and steadfast and one which enters within the veil, where Jesus has entered as a forerunner for us."

Who drags an anchor to the desert, to a land of endless days without rain? To a hard-packed and heat-drenched place? To a forgetting place? To a place where the Evil Whisperer questions God's power, His compassion?

I pick up that anchor, that hope. I throw it out, toward the sound of rain. It is not a hope resting in doctors, in treatment plans, or in the number of days. It is hope based on Someone who stood with those He loved at the edge of a grave and faced death.

This hope sails out—beyond the veil of dust, the veil of this life—until it anchors into eternity, the reality yet seen where Christ has already gone to prepare the way.

This is where I pin my hope—to a life beyond this life. A place where my dad says his real life will begin.

Hope does not end there.

Here is the mystery. I throw the anchor that fastens into eternity where Christ is seated, yet Jesus is also with me in the desert as an anchor of hope on this side.

He stands beside me, back at the bench, under the eaves, where I listen to the rain.

He is the promise of water in desert places. The lifeboat in tsunami seasons. The shield when you are left hanging in a lightning storm. The refuge when haboobs swoop from one mile high. Limitless water when you forget to pack enough. A lifeline when the doctor says there are no more options. He is the anchor on both sides of eternity. He is the answer to the doubts raised by the Evil Whisperer, because Jesus is God, all power. God, all compassion.

Jesus is hope.

"Do you believe this?" Jesus asked Martha at the tomb of her brother (John 11:26). He had listened to Martha, and then Jesus had a question of His own. "Do you believe this?" At the edge of a grave you discover what you believe. Or Who.

He asks me the same question. "Do you believe this?"

Do I believe this as I stand near a grave? Do I believe this as the life of someone I love hangs in the balance? Do I believe this as I gaze into the face of God with my questions? My anger? Do I believe this as I fall prostrate at His feet?

Do I believe?

Twelve

The Narrow Place

My camera lens captures the beauty of boulders balancing on boulders and of natural tunnels and rock faces polished smooth by countless years of rushing water from the monsoon rains. Rocks appear to be the best thing growing in this area of South Mountain, along the National Trail. I hear, but do not see, a rock wren as he trills his morning greetings from a nearby crevice. I keep a watchful eye for rattlers. Last week I encountered a snake sunning himself, his midsection wide from a morning meal.

I hike under azure skies, the orange flame of ocotillo in full bloom. Mollie's pink tongue hangs long as she flops flat, panting on a sun-drenched trail, tired from her adventures in the underbrush. It's a Crayola day, the colors vibrant.

I reach my destination, a slim opening guarded by a lone mesquite tree, the bark rough with age. Two gigantic boulders rise from the fine gravel floor and loom above me, leaving a twelve-inch passage. I attempt the narrow way with full equipment, but my water hydration pack wedges in the tiny passageway. Mollie whines, unsure what to do. I try again, backpack removed. I shimmy my body sideways along the smooth granite, sucking in my breath. It's a tight squeeze. I whistle for Mollie to follow.

Fat Man's Pass has room for only one.

———

In high school, I was on the cross-country team. The races always began with a mass start—everyone lined up in a group; faster runners jockeyed for the lead starting positions. At the sound of the gun we took off, seven varsity racers for each school, our feet pounding beneath us.

Our team ran in pairs—strength in numbers—a trick our coach taught us to psych out the other team. She encouraged us to use strategy when running the race—especially when passing. She trained us to pass the competition while running uphill, not down—which was expected—as part of the mental game of proving strength and fitness.

Although we started the race in a group and ran the course in pairs, once we approached the finish line, it was every runner for herself. The finish line was laid out with barricades, cones, or rope to form a chute, where only one runner could pass through at a time, leaving no argument on the order of finishers.

We had to pass through a narrow place in order to finish. There was room for only one.

———

Dad's world is narrowing, as his life journey is ending, but it is not the first time his way has narrowed as he faced eternal choices. It's not the first time he has faced death. In a narrow place, years ago, Dad encountered Jesus.

Every year when I was a child, our family of six traveled to northern Wisconsin for Christmas vacation to spend time in Solon Springs, where Dad was born and raised. Avid snowmobilers, we anticipated long hours riding on the groomed forest trails.[1]

The year I was fifteen, Dad and my brother, Phil, took two snowmobiles out for a trial run. The ground was covered with two inches of fresh powder on a cold, clear, thirty-eight-degrees-below-zero morning. Dad headed east into the sun on a field road he'd driven hundreds of times both as an adult and, decades earlier, as a boy bringing the cows back and forth from the barn.

In no time, Dad had the snowmobile floating along at sixty miles per hour. Dad was in complete control—man over machine.

With the end of the road approaching, Dad decelerated to forty-five. He did not see the two strands of barbed wire, temporarily placed across the road to keep a horse from getting into the woods during deer season. Dad found himself in the snow, his snowmobile seventy-five feet up the trail, still running.

What had happened?

Dad stood, only to fall back down. Only then did he discover the barbed wire wrapped around his head and deeply embedded in his throat. The blood on his glove convinced him that he had severed his jugular vein. That he was dying.

He whispered, "No. Jesus, no."

The prayer surprised him. Rather than being neat and thought out, it was spoken as if talking to a friend. Peace enveloped him. The profuse bleeding stopped. Dad unwound the barbed wire from his head, panicking when the last section of wire wouldn't come out. The wire stuck. Deep.

Dad heard the whir of my brother's snowmobile and a new fear gripped him.

"God, Phil mustn't hit the fence."

Dad stood to warn my brother, but the wire jerked Dad off his feet. He lay in the snow, sobbing, "Help me, Jesus." Dad tipped his head way back. He felt the gash open and was able to pull the wire out. He stood and waved, stopping Phil in time.

One glance at Phil's frightened face sent Dad stumbling for his snowmobile. Uncontrollable panic seized Dad as he squeezed the hammer tight against the handlebar. With Phil following close behind on his own snowmobile, Dad flew down the road, past the sawmill, through the gate, past the barn, and into the front yard. He rode like one possessed. Dad leapt off the back of the still rolling machine and ran for the house. In the entrance he felt the peace of Jesus again.

"You can't go in there like this," he told himself. "Your wife, three daughters, and elderly parents are in there. Get control of yourself."

Dad calmly opened the kitchen door and walked to the sink. He told Mom he was badly hurt and not to faint. Mom assessed the damage, covered his gaping wounds with a washcloth, and asked my uncle to drive them thirty miles to the hospital, a torturous ride where Dad felt every tar strip and frost boil. Radiating pain shot up his neck, making him unable to suppress a groan and causing him to wonder if he had broken something in his spine when he was jerked off the machine.

Mom sang Scripture songs, melodies taken from sections of the Bible, her head on Dad's shoulder, her hand keeping Dad's head locked against hers. "They that wait upon the Lord shall renew their strength," Mom sang. "They shall mount up with wings as eagles."[2] Again, the pain and panic subsided.

It took three layers of stitches, fifty-seven in all, to mend the damage. Dad's tongue was lacerated and he lost four teeth. The barbs scratched his trachea but missed his jugular vein by a fraction of a millimeter. The surgeon touched the tip of his surgical instrument to indicate how close Dad had been to bleeding out.

Dad always pointed to that experience as the day he encountered God personally, when he knew God loved him without question. Before that day Dad had known Bible stories from years in church, but he struggled seriously with his faith. He was ready to give it up unless Jesus met him in a real way.

All other options narrowed for him, as he encountered God in a snowbank. Jesus gave him back his life, and Dad turned his focus to follow Him.

Thirty-seven years later, the way has narrowed again.

———

When the doctor called to say the cancer had moved to Dad's brain and a seven-millimeter tumor had shown up on the MRI, Mom had to take the message. Dad was out on the tractor clearing the driveway from the latest blizzard.

In my childhood memories, I picture Dad after each snowstorm, driving his Allis-Chalmers tractor, clearing the way before the county vehicles arrived to plow the road leading to my parents' home, four miles out of town.

Dad tried to show me how to start the tractor once, no key, only a complicated series of clutches and levers, with a stick in the fuel tank to check the level of gas. I couldn't do it.

Dad still drives the same 1949 tractor. He bundles up against the elements and meticulously removes the snow, making the way clear. The last time I was back, he fired up the old orange lady so the great-grandkids could take a spin with their parents around the property, thrilling the hearts of toddlers who had no clue to the significance of the ride.

Memories of the tractor, my dad, and the farm are inseparable.

When Dad came in from plowing, Mom told him the doctor's report. Dad said, "It's just another bump in the road."

This is a man who understands bumps and stones, hard ground and snow, and other obstacles that need to be removed. He's been doing it his entire life, out on his tractor, while the snow was still falling—clearing the road.

Perhaps the knowledge came on another country road when blood stained the newly fallen snow and then stained a seeping washcloth held to a neck with gaping wounds or while Mom sang songs and peace descended on a bumpy road as they raced to the hospital. Maybe the purpose of bumps, barbed wired, and obstacles in the road is to bring us face-to-face with the One who loves us most. And once there, we realize we are not alone on the bumpiest journeys.

"I will live until I die, and then my real life will begin," Dad says. Death—the final bump in the road. In reality, death is only another obstacle to be removed, to make the way clear.

The thud alerts me where I stand guard outside the men's bathroom at a store in Albert Lea.

"Dad? Do you need help?"

"Go get your mother."

I inch the door open. Dad is sprawled on the grimy tile. His legs block me from opening the door wider.

The tumors have multiplied in Dad's brain and on his spinal column. The doctors have given their prediction on number of days. Dad has lost the use of his left arm. His legs give out without warning—not only in town, but later that night at their home while Mom gets him ready for bed.

"I'm dying," he says to Mom as she tries to help him to his feet. "Is this how it goes?"

"We've had fifty-five great years together," Mom says.

"Too short," Dad sobs. "It was too short."

They hold each other and weep on the floor of the bedroom they have shared for five decades.

The next day Dad is out with his walker supervising projects being completed on the property. The convertible comes out for a spin. He climbs the windmill to check the blades. Mom watches from the kitchen window, heart in her throat, but says when I question this decision, "What is the worst that can happen?"

Dad is facing the finish line of his faith. The hardest reality for him is not facing his own finish line, but leaving my mom to finish her race without him. They have always run as a pair, even sharing cancer together.

"I don't want your mom to be a widow," Dad says to me. "I see the widows sitting together at church. I don't want that for your mother."

I suddenly understand the extra tests and treatments Dad chose to do, even when there was little hope. I clear my throat. Swallow hard. "Isn't there a verse about God being a husband for the widow?" I ask.[3] I let my voice tease, although I am struggling with control. "After you are gone, Mom gets Jesus."

Getting Jesus. Ever since that day in the snowbank, Dad has been content with that.

The strength of Dad's physical body is weakening. His spiritual focus is clarifying as he loses more and more of the earthly bonds that restrain him.

His eyes focus on his destination. He is in the narrow place. Matthew 7:13 states, "You can enter God's Kingdom only through the narrow gate" (NLT). The narrow gate—where there is room for only one.

Yet Dad is not alone. In a cross-country race, each runner finishes individually, but in the journey of faith, Jesus promises He will be there at the beginning and the end. He is there for all of life's bumps on the road. "Let us lay aside every weight, and the sin which so easily ensnares us, and let us run with endurance the race that is set before us, looking unto Jesus, the author and finisher of our faith" (Heb. 12:1–2 NKJV). When Dad cried out to Him from a bloody snowbank, Jesus was there. And now at the end?

Jesus.

Thirteen

The Final Solo

"Would you like to sort through the last of Dad's classroom books?" Mom asks a group of us one afternoon as we sit at the dining room table.

Dad is napping in his chair.

"Sure!" We welcome the diversion.

We drag in four musty boxes from the garage and spread them all around. My eyes widen at the treasure.

My dad always loved a good story. As a ninth-grade English teacher, Dad read out loud to his students for more than three decades. He continued the tradition of his mother, who read to the family after the milking and chores were done as they sat around the table at the conclusion of the evening meal. My dad's parents were both sticklers for education, Grandpa because he didn't go to school past the eighth grade and Grandma because she was an elementary school teacher.

Dad kept a lending library in his classroom, books he collected throughout the years. Occasionally he would bring a book home, telling me I should read it. One book, *Mr. and Mrs. Bo Jo Jones*, was about two teenagers who fell in love in high school, had sex the night of prom, and ended up with an unplanned pregnancy. That was the only "talk" my dad had with me about sexuality. I think I was thirteen. He let a story do the teaching.

Another time he handed me the book *Christy* by Catherine Marshall, the fictional story of a young woman with a heart for God who went to teach school in Cutter Cap in the Appalachian Mountains. With 576 pages, it was a challenge for a ten-year-old girl to read, but that book has remained a favorite story to this day. *Christy* did more for establishing my worldview on compassion and loving others than any nonfiction book on the subject.

I learned those truths through story.

Jesus was known as a great storyteller. People liked to ask Him questions. In fact, the Bible records 183 of those queries. According to author Philip Yancey, with all the questions people asked Him, Jesus might have become known as the great answerer. But that's not what happened. He answered only a few of those questions. The rest of the time, He sat down and told a story.[1]

"A certain man had two sons"[2] . . . "two men went up into the temple to pray"[3] . . . "a certain man was going down from Jerusalem to Jericho; and fell among robbers."[4]

Jesus told truth through story.

"Take what you want," Mom says as we sort through the boxes. The carpet is covered with old paperbacks and worn classics.

Two nieces divide my dad's collection of Mark Twain. Our youngest son, Zach, takes *Cry the Beloved Country*, his favorite story from high school, set in 1940s South Africa. My daughter Katelyn and my nephew, both history majors, gladly keep the old newspapers from Kennedy's assassination and from the first men on the moon. Our daughter Aleah, an ancient Greek major, takes *The Odyssey* and *Dialogues of Plato*. My daughter-in-law, Rachel, emails to request several classics. She reminds me she lost her entire book collection when her parents' house burned down when she was in college, including her collection of Nancy Drew. I pull twelve Nancy Drew books and add them to the pile.

Since news of Dad's diagnosis, former students have sent Dad cards and notes. Several students mention how Dad gave spelling tests every week. He told his students if everyone in the class scored 100 percent on the test, he would stand on his head. On his desk. In his thirty-five years of teaching, I think he only did it once. For years he practiced at home on the living room carpet to make sure he still could do it.

One of his former students jotted this note in a card:

> Hi Mr Hankins! You gave me a wonderful gift when you read Ol' Yeller to us in class and cried at the end. Every night 'til my boys were 12, I read to them before bed. When we got to a sad part in the book, I'd just let myself cry and kept reading. You helped me to give my two boys empathy. Thank you so much.

I cannot find a copy of *Old Yeller*, but I do find two other books Dad read to his classes: *Merchant of Venice* and *Passage to India*. The books are filled with Dad's handwritten notes in the margins. *Passage to India* also includes a heart with the names of my parents ("Stanley Loves Lois") inside the front cover. I choose the doodled volume as a reminder of the love story I have witnessed for half a century.

Home is where our stories begin. It is within the family relationships we first live out plot and trouble and theme. I have learned important truths while living in family. I have also learned important truths from the books I have read on my journey, stories told by Jesus, and books collected by my dad. "[God] has spoken the Alpha, knows the day he will shout the Omega," author Adam McHugh writes, "and our present lives are engaged in listening for the rest of his letters."[5]

As we sort through the last tomes in the cardboard boxes, I can't help but hope my children will continue the tradition as they read their grandfather's books. I hope they will remember the man who loved a good story, but who also remained a teacher through this final chapter, who heard the Alpha cry after a snowmobile accident and spent his life listening for God's other letters.

The fact that we are in the Omega chapter is no surprise to us, but the nearing to the final page is difficult. At times—agony. I want to tuck the book back on the shelf.

When I was a teenager, I went through a stage when I would skip ahead to read the last page of a book. For whatever reason, I couldn't stand the suspense and had to discover how the story ended. Then I went back and finished reading the book from where I left off, but from the viewpoint of knowing the ending.

In essence, I was then reading the story backward. The last page gave me the completed picture of the drama and character development found in earlier pages of the story. If the book was a mystery, the last page told me "who done it." If the book was a romance, I discovered on the final page if the hero and heroine ended up living happily ever after.

Last pages unveil the culmination of a story being told by the writer.

In His stories, Jesus taught that the two parts of a person—the inner and outer life—are inseparable. Looking good on the outside is not enough. True character is unveiled through what we do. "We can read backward from our actions into our hearts," Mark Labberton writes.[6]

Our final actions are, in essence, the last page.

As much as I want to avoid reading my dad's final page, he has been writing the words before my eyes. If I could read his life backward, I would find the clues to his last page by actions I have witnessed all his life.

Dad saves his most valuable lesson for the end: how to face eternity without fear.

Dad shuffles to the front of the church, the sanctuary of faith in this farming community where he has lived for half a century.

His feet drag as he pushes the walker one-handed. His left arm swings uselessly next to his body; his limbs communicate a story all their own.

Mom gets a glass of water and places it next to his good side. Radiation has destroyed his mouth's ability to make saliva, and the tumors in his brain have begun to affect his vocal cords, yet the teller of stories has one final tale to tell.

"I checked the obituaries this morning," Dad quips. "I'm not dead yet."

The congregation laughs. Hesitantly. Dad has asked to speak to his neighbors and friends, a Last Lecture type of thing, after my sister Renae encouraged him to share his final thoughts and blessings for those he will leave behind.[7]

Dad sings a chorus of a praise hymn, thanking the Lord for saving him.

I grab the first Kleenex.

Dad thanks God, thanks his friends, and thanks my mom.

"Thank you for over fifty-five years as my helpmate. I should be taking care of you because of your health issues, but I can't even put on my own shirt."

I grab a second Kleenex.

For twenty-five minutes my dad spins stories and tells jokes, starring his favorite Norwegian rascals, Sven and Ole.

"Ole was puttering in the yard when here came Sven walking up the road pulling a big log chain. 'Sven, all week you've been pulling that chain up the road. What's up?'

"'Of course I'm pulling it. Have you ever tried pushin' a chain?'"

Dad takes a sip of water. His hand shakes.

"Lately, I've been guilty of pushing that cancer chain to no avail."

Dad is a weaver of tales. Some of my earliest memories are of him sitting at the table at my grandparents' home, holding a circle of people in the palm of his hand. With his words. Even after two and a half years of battling cancer, he has not lost the gift.

Dad has never been afraid of tears, I remind myself as I grab another Kleenex.

Dad ends his talk by singing the song about God watching over sparrows, the song his dad, my grandfather, sang when he milked the cows.

> Why should I feel discouraged? Why should the shadows come?
> Why should my heart be lonely? And cry for heaven and home?
> When Jesus is my portion; my constant friend is He.
> For His eye is on the sparrow and I know He watches me.
> His eye is on the sparrow and I know He watches me.[8]

I grab a fourth Kleenex.

Years ago my brother got Dad a shirt emblazoned with the words *Real Men Sing Loud*. The real man part is still true. The loud part? His voice is raspy and broken. It cracks on the high notes. It's not the strong tenor I remember. Cancer attempts to silence my dad's song.

But not today.

Victory songs are not always about volume. When Dad's voice fails, the congregation joins in, one by one. First, a white-haired lady in the third row joins in, tentatively at first, but then with more volume. A young mom jostling a toddler joins the chorus, blending in with a soothing alto. A teenage boy slouched in the back row sits a little straighter and comes in for the last few lines. Friends and neighbors turn Dad's solo into an unrehearsed ensemble, proving victory songs aren't about singing alone.

> I sing because I'm happy. I sing because I'm free.
> For His eye is on the sparrow, and I know He watches me.
> His eye is on the sparrow, and I know He watches me.[9]

The final note fades away. "That's all I've got," Dad says. He shuffles back to his seat.

Later, when we get home, Dad mentions he forgot to say some sentences he wanted to share. He wonders if he delivered his message in the way he wanted.

We assure him he did great. "You made us laugh. You made us cry. And you made us sing," we tell him.

What more could a storyteller want?

Fourteen

Sunrise, Sunset

Several years before cancer touched our family's story, Kevin and I joined a group of twenty-seven, including chaperones and teens from a Phoenix children's home, for a quick presunrise photo at the trailhead of South Kaibab before a fifteen-mile hike in and out of the Grand Canyon. Cameras flashed in the darkness. The more experienced hikers reminded novices to eat and drink before they became hungry and thirsty to keep the lactic acid from building up in their legs. Last-minute stops were made at the outhouse, backpacks were strapped in place; we began the descent, my husband and I in the role of sweepers.

Five million people visit the Grand Canyon each year, most content to take the shuttle buses to various scenic lookouts, snap photos, and leave with a sense they have seen everything—the layers of rock, a sunrise, and maybe a condor flying overhead. Photographer Kathleeen Jo Ryan writes of a different world that awaits those who step over the edge: "From the South Rim, the experience is orderly, almost antiseptic, and does not require risk or effort. There are paved turnouts and neatly organized guard rails. . . . The Canyon I have come to love appears forbidding, barren, hostile . . . and beyond my reach. The magnitude numbs and I am lost in a sea of insignificance."[1]

We were about to join the minority, those who step off the rim into the inner canyon as participants, no longer satisfied to be detached observers.

The early morning dusk provided enough light that we did not need our headlamps on the switchbacks through the Kaibab limestone, the crowning rock layer of the canyon. Those planning to run the canyon, "rabbits" we called them, soon left us in their dust. I hoped they would remember to eat and drink or, I knew from past experience, we would catch them later. The story "The Tortoise and the Hare" is especially relevant when hiking the Grand Canyon.

Dawn was lightening the inner walls when we reached Cedar Ridge, one and a half miles from the top. A peek over the edge provided views of both sides of the ridge, rock layers stacked like dishes—Coconino Sandstone, Hermit Shale, Esplanade Sandstone, Redwall Limestone. In the Grand Canyon, "time is measured in geology."[2] We snapped several photos in the magical gold of a new sunrise.

By the time we reached Skeleton Point, three miles from the start, we could see our first view of the Colorado River, a thin serpentine ribbon that appeared miles in the distance. We had hiked down two thousand feet in elevation and had another twenty-six hundred feet more to drop. An older member of the group was already struggling with a painful right knee.

Rangers advised turning around at Skeleton Point for a moderate day hike. Signs everywhere warned of not doing what we were about to do—descend to the Colorado and hike back out all in the same day.

I stopped to take photos of a claret cup cactus, the vibrant red bloom showing bright in the surrounding rock. I snapped pictures of the orange blossoms of a globe mallow and the pale lavender petals of a sego lily. Surrounded by indescribable magnificence, I found relief in the small and intricate. The surrounding rock layers spoke a story of strength, but I discovered solace in the fragile.

With 1,771 different categorized plants in the Grand Canyon,[3] I could take plant photos all day, but like other travelers, the layered rock soon captured me. As the sun rose, the beams hit deeper into the canyon, highlighting the stacking layers. Red. Umber. Bronze. Sienna. My eyes absorbed it all until I was intoxicated with color.

The last mile of descent was brutal on our joints. With the exception of practice hikes to put miles on the legs, there wasn't an exercise in existence that could prepare the body for the constant pounding. We struggled with pain, but the older chaperone was in the worst shape, leaning heavily on his trekking sticks. Our pace slowed to a crawl. My husband and I shook our heads and sent secret eye messages. *We should have made him turn back at Skeleton Point.* We knew from experience the most difficult part was in front of us. We also knew each hour descending meant at least double on the ascent. We glanced at our watches. *Ouch.*

The Grand Canyon poses a mental and physical challenge not experienced in other hiking, the majority of which is done in mountains. When a hiker gets tired hiking a mountain, they can simply turn around, immediately getting relief by going downhill. Canyon hiking is exactly the opposite. The most intense workout is the ascent, when the body and legs are already compromised.

As we began the climb up the Bright Angel Trail, we met a woman collapsed on the ground. She had slipped on a small puddle, her fully loaded pack sending her sprawling at an awkward angle.

Her leg was broken.

We rigged up a piece of shade using a raincoat, rope, and hiking sticks to provide relief from the hot sun. We sent the older chaperone ahead, knowing he would need every minute possible to hike out, while we waited with the woman. Another hiker ran back several miles to get a ranger.

We dug out pain meds from our first aid kit and eased off the woman's boot. She had planned to meet two friends for a week of camping. She worried how to get a message to them or to her husband back in Phoenix. Two hours passed while we chitchatted and her leg swelled. The ranger arrived and explained that the woman would be transported to the river on a spinal board, rafted across to a landing site, and then helicoptered out. The ranger thanked us, but said he had everything under control.

We ascended at a fast clip, figuring everyone would be waiting for us at the summit. Four miles later, we met the chaperone and several teens at Indian Gardens, resting in the shaded coolness. The rabbits—their legs full of lactic acid—had not heeded the warning to eat and drink. They had "hit the wall," reaching the mental and physical point where their bodies no longer wanted to keep moving, almost as if their energy levels had washed down the drain. We prodded them along and began the remaining 4.8-mile climb. The trail became a wicked taskmaster, taunting our muscles and providing a lesson in character building.

My husband and I told jokes, repeated stories, played mind games, anything to keep the group moving. We met hikers walking down, laughing and skipping, unaware our fates soon awaited them once they turned around. The rabbits' gaits deteriorated even further, a stiff-legged Frankenstein walk of utter misery. We sought relief in the shade of rock overhangs, but mostly we toughed out the heat, hoping each passing switchback would be the last.

Near dusk, we took our last step out of the inner canyon and onto the upper rim. No one could question if we qualified as active participants in experiencing the canyon—predawn at the trailhead, sunrise over Cedar Ridge, wildflowers, the lady with the broken leg, and tales of wretchedness on the switchbacks.

As we loaded into vans, teens who reached the summit hours earlier showed me sunset photos on their cameras—the sky aflame with color amid darkened silhouettes, an event I had missed in the single-minded focus of crawling out of the canyon. I compared the shots to my sunrise photos from earlier in the day. Yellows versus oranges. Golds versus brilliant reds. Sunrise. Sunset. The beauty of both left me breathless.

Sometimes the only difference is the direction you are facing. Are you in the coming? Are you in the going?

———

It is one thing to read about the end of life, to observe death from a distance. It is another to participate in the dying, with someone you love, in the difficult beauty. As a family, we step over the edge of the rim on Dad's journey. We try to prepare ourselves, emotionally and spiritually, but we find ourselves "hitting the wall," as we struggle to stay engaged when our bodies and brains want to shut down. The most difficult beautiful remains.

I stay in Minnesota as long as possible but find myself having to choose between two stories. Do I stay with Dad or return to Arizona for Zach's high school graduation? I have never wanted more to be a clone. I pack my suitcase and hug my dad in the entryway to the kitchen, but technically I should call it the exitway, because I am heading to the airport.

"I love you." I want to shout it loud, but it gets trapped somewhere in my throat, where my heart has taken residence, and it comes out in a strangled whisper. "I'll see you later." I turn back, one more time, to peer over my shoulder, and watch Dad shuffle into the house to rest in his favorite chair.

He is in too much pain to come to say good-bye at the airport.

A few hours later, I put my suitcase down so I can hug my mom with both arms as she thanks me for coming. I can hardly bear the thought that I need to catch a plane.

"I love you," we both say, and I pray for at least a thousand more days to whisper the words. Before I enter the airport, I turn back and watch her get into her car.

"I'll see you later," I say to the departing taillights.

I'll see you later. A casual way of parting. When the children were little, we'd say, "See you later, alligator." In Spanish the words are *hasta luego*. I have always liked the phrase. It is a way of saying good-bye without actually uttering that word.

"I'll see you later" holds the promise of tomorrow, a promise when hours of time are gained, not lost. We will enter timelessness, the promise of continual "See you laters" and continual tomorrows.

A timelessness without pain, without cancer, without good-byes and strangled words and swallowing back sobs in the airport bathroom.

The promise of later.

Here is our hope. Here is the beauty in the difficult, in the impossible. The Author *has* written a different ending. It is the in-between that is hard.

I am leaving life and death in Minnesota, the precious coming and going. I am returning to graduation events for our youngest, the ending of his high school experience and the beginning of his life as an adult. The ending. The beginning. The daily rhythm of the rising and the setting. And the sometimes difficult in-between.

"We live our lives in between the dying and the rising. We have not fully experienced the dying. Nor have we lived the fullness of the risen life. We linger somewhere in between," Macrina Wiederkehr writes.[4]

Dad is in the time of in-between, but his space is narrowing, as he is closer than ever to the rising, the promise of our faith, where he will be fully grasped by Christ. We are the ones who hold tightly as we watch him let go of more and more so he can gain Jesus. We are surrounded by the difficult beautiful.

In the course of one month, Dad goes from using a cane to a walker, from a walker to a wheelchair, and from a wheelchair to a hospital bed in the living room. A bedside commode. A Hoyer lift. Oxygen tanks.

My parents' Bible study group of more than thirty-five years meets on their regular night, except now they gather next to Dad's bed. Dad mostly sleeps while they sing worship songs and share prayer requests like they have done throughout the decades. Real men cry real tears as they say their good-byes, their hearts holding to an unseen reality. A final song is sung and a friend comments, "This. This is how I want to leave this earth. With friends and family singing at my bedside."

Through it all, Mom takes care of Dad. She sleeps on the couch to be available if he needs her. She gives him meds. She touches him every time she passes the bed. Each night Dad and Mom end the day as they have for many years—with love, prayer, devotions, and a good-night kiss.

Beautiful.

Difficult.

I speak with Dad one last time. I tell him the details of the upcoming graduation. Dad interrupts my story to pray a blessing over my son in a quiet, stumbling voice.

"Father, thank You for my grandson. Thank You for the favor over his life."

The veil separating our two worlds is lifting. At least for Dad. I don't want the call to end, but I can tell Dad is tired. Fading.

"I love you, Dad."

"I love you too. I wish I could love you longer, but I don't think . . ."

"But you get to go to heaven."

"Yeah, a good thing."

Later that day he slips into a coma.

Mom, constantly at Dad's side, whispers it is okay to go to heaven to be with Jesus. She lays her head on Dad's chest and weeps her "See you laters."

I am not with Dad when he dies. My mom and sister Lisa, who are among those at his bedside, comment on the peacefulness of his passing. No drama. No struggle. One final breath.

Breath.

One of the last conditions that holds us to this world.

I remember when our oldest son, Nate, was born. There were difficulties in his birth, and his skin was blue in the brief seconds I saw him before the doctor whisked him behind a screen. No newly born, on-the-mommy's-tummy photos for me.

In the agonizing seconds that followed, I waited. And listened. Soon there was a breath and a wail. The final forming of our son was complete.

He left behind the safety of the womb and breathed himself into an entirely new world, no longer living in amniotic security.

Genesis 2:7 says, "God formed man of dust from the ground, and breathed into his nostrils the breath of life; and man became a living being."

All other created beings were spoken into existence: dogs, giraffes, palm trees, the sun, the planets, butterflies, whales. Only man was personally formed and then breathed to life. A face-to-face, cheek-to-cheek, breath-to-breath creating.

From One who loves.

The word *formed* is repeated in Psalm 139:13, "For You formed my inward parts; You wove me in my mother's womb." The psalmist continues in verse 16, "Your eyes have seen my unformed substance; and in Your book were all written the days that were ordained for me, when as yet there was not one of them." God continues the forming of life beyond the borders of the Garden of Eden. He does some of His best work in secret, in the confines of a woman's womb.

God then gives the crowning miracle—breath. If you have ever witnessed a birth and the exchange of one world to the next with the gasp of that first breath, you know what I'm talking about. Job 12:9–10 says, "Who among all these does not know that the hand of the LORD has done this, in whose hand is the life of every living thing, and the breath of all mankind?"

"Your breath is not your own; it has been borrowed from God,"[5] Wiederkehr writes, and so on the completion of his days, my dad no longer needed God's borrowed breath. When Dad's breath returned to his Creator, the last thing holding him to this earth was gone. He was free to leave this world for a new one.

"Take a good look at God's wonders—they'll take your breath away" (Ps. 66:5 Message).

Sunrise. Sunset. Dad is birthed into breathless eternity.

Fifteen

The Bigger Shadow

After a standing-room-only funeral filled with stories and tears and jokes about heaven getting louder, we bury Dad's ashes in Solon Springs, Wisconsin, next to the graves of his parents and grandparents.

"Stop the car!" I tell Mom after the service when we pass a grove of pine trees that I recognize from another day, years ago, when I photographed Dad standing under the trees.

Mom pulls the car over on the shoulder of a busy roadway. Campers and RVs speed around us, the drivers shaking their heads, believing we are crazy tourists.

"I want to take a picture," I say.

We brush aside knee-high grass and purple bellflowers as we walk closer to the forest. I pose with arms wide in the shadow of full-grown evergreens.

I need the reminder of towering pines.

Six decades ago, when Dad was sixteen, he and his high school classmates planted the trees, acres and acres, for the Mosinee Paper Company. Most of them saved the money they earned—seventy-five cents an hour—for spring prom.

Sometimes when we find ourselves doing something to earn money, it is good to look around and ask, "Am I planting something that will outlast my life?"

———

After returning home from Dad's funeral, I begin to experience troubling physical symptoms. Numerous appointments with my gynecologist and oncologist result in genetic testing, an ultrasound, and a biopsy.

"I think you should consider a hysterectomy," my gynecologist says, echoing the words of the oncologist I saw the day before.

"The biopsy was negative." I try to close the conversation, along with the front of my paper gown, as I sit on the edge of the exam table. The room is decorated with Harley Davidson décor, complete with photos of my doctor riding his favorite motorcycle. I like the fact that my doctor understands the need to escape the confines of four walls.

"You are anemic from blood loss. It's possible you have developed endometrial cancer from your medication." The doctor refers to an estrogen blocker I have been taking since I completed treatment, a medication designed to keep the estrogen-eating breast cancer from returning. The doctor assures me that endometrial cancer is a rare side effect. Given the circumstances, I don't find his words comforting, preferring to use the word *rare* in front of words like *diamond* or *painting*.

"The ultrasound came back clean," I remind him. Was I really hearing the C-word again?

"Your mom's ovarian diagnosis also concerns me. It is a silent killer."

This stops me. I am also concerned with Mom's diagnosis. I know breast cancer and ovarian cancer can be genetically linked. But seriously? A possible second cancer for me?

"I'm going to Peru." The exam room walls shrink inward as the shadow lengthens.

"Schedule the surgery after you return home."

I numbly put on my clothes before going to the appointment desk. Was this some kind of sick joke? Doesn't our family even get a few months' reprieve? Could I have inherited more than brown eyes from my mom? Could I possibly be facing the shadow of cancer again?

Kevin and I pack our bags for Peru. The shadow climbs into my luggage and makes it through security, despite my efforts to compartmentalize him into an I-will-deal-with-this-when-I-get-home place in my mind. One of the stops on our itinerary is the city of Arequipa. We arrive at six in the morning after an all-night bus ride from Cusco. After we settle into our hostel, we walk the few blocks to the downtown plaza.

The volcano is impossible to miss.

Located twelve miles outside the city, as a condor flies, the volcano dominates the landscape. The name of the volcano sounds like a cast-off from a B-grade movie script: El Misti.

Legend says the indigenous people, the Aymara, first gave Arequipa its name, *ari* meaning "peak" and *quipa* meaning "lying behind." Arequipa, the place that lies behind the peak.[1]

In essence, the city exists beneath the shadow of a mountain, a volcano. Arequipa is a city constructed beneath shadow. El Misti last erupted from 1450 to 1470, yet it continues to have seismic activity, most recently in August 2012, when 224 earthquakes were registered. The experts were quick to reassure the public that no eruption was imminent, but the volcano was "waking up" and could no longer be considered dormant.[2] Because of the proximity to Peru's second largest city, as well as its history, El Misti is considered one of the world's most dangerous volcanoes.[3]

What is it like to live near a waking mountain? To dwell beneath shadow?

I live with the shadow of cancer.

Standing in the shadow of the volcano and still grieving Dad's death, I fear I will never escape the diagnosis. At times I feel it pursues me. The shadow of cancer looms on my landscape. It is easy for me to think, *Let's face it, cancer will eventually kill me.*

Author and cancer survivor Lynn Eib understands the shadow: "I tried various methods to get rid of cancer's shadow. I closed my eyes very tightly. *I don't see any shadow.* But it was very hard to go through a normal day with my eyes closed. I got very busy. *The shadow won't be able to catch up with me.* But shadows are much faster than I realized. I thought positive. *That's not a shadow. It's a big, happy, black balloon!* But it sure was dark under there."[4]

Eyes closed. Busyness. Thinking positive. I have tried them all, but I have discovered the same thing. It is still dark under here. Very dark.

One of the best-known psalms, Psalm 23, has King David declaring that even when he walks in the shadow of death, he will not be afraid. I find myself facing again the fragileness of my mortality. The limits of my own humanness. Unlike David, I am afraid. I find myself struggling in the shadow of not being in control.

That night in Arequipa, Kevin and I enjoy a bowl of quinoa soup on a balcony café, three stories above the city while an entertainer plays music on a pan flute, a traditional Peruvian instrument. The haunting notes of a love song barely fade away before the musician starts a 1960s song by Simon and Garfunkel: "The Sound of Silence." I hum a line from the song, about the darkness being a friend. I stop. Has darkness somehow become my friend? My familiar companion? I shudder. The last thing I want is the shadow of cancer to be a familiar friend.

Can I sever my ties to the shadow? To the darkness spoken over my life?

I am heart weary of the shadow of cancer that dogs my steps. How do I escape? David says that even in death—the ultimate fragile, human, uncontrollable place—he is not afraid. How is that possible?

Perhaps the answer can be found in the shadow of a volcano.

———

We climb into a beat-up four-wheel-drive vehicle for our two-hour trip to El Misti. After a labyrinth of dirt roads through the Salinas and Aguada Blanca National Reserve, our guide pulls over. Three vicuñas, South American camelids highly prized for their wool, are grazing in the mountain's shadow.

At a Peruvian market the day before, the sellers all guaranteed the local textiles we examined were genuine alpaca and not cheap imitations. Not knowledgeable in yarn origin and quality, I examined the product carefully to see if a small alpaca tag, guaranteeing authenticity, was sewn into the corner. At all the little shops and road stands we perused, however, no seller ever claimed to be selling the valuable vicuña wool.

Vicuñas—endangered animals, once poached nearly to extinction—are allowed to be captured once every three years in a government-sanctioned *chacu*, a community event where villagers work together to herd the animals so they can be sheared. According to our guide, the vicuñas are then returned to the wild, ensuring their protection. At an exclusive shop in Arequipa the day before, I had fingered a fashionable vicuña scarf with a price tag of $1,500.

As I try to photograph the illusive and timid vicuñas in their natural habitat in the Andes, I find myself angling my camera, trying to get the best photo. My plan is to position the shot so the animals are in the foreground, with the mountain behind them, but I can't manage a good photo with the position of the sun. Even as an amateur photographer, I understand shadows fall opposite their light source. The sun and the shadows are not cooperating.

Which is the way of shadows. A shadow is in front, if the sun is behind, and vice versa.

Perhaps this explains David's ability to walk in the shadow and not be afraid. "Even though I walk through the valley of the shadow of death, I fear no evil," David writes, "for You are with me" (Ps. 23:4). Why wasn't David afraid? Because his eyes were on the One he was facing, not on the shadow. Turned toward the Light, the shadow fell behind him, out of view. It was a matter of perspective, a matter of which way he faced.

Once David found himself no longer focusing on the shadow but on the One who loved him most, he was able to embrace a different shadow. "He who dwells in the shelter of the Most High will abide in the shadow of the Almighty," writes David in Psalm 91:1.

David learned to live under a bigger shadow—the shadow of the almighty God.

This shadow is safe and protective. This shadow is not one of fear, but of trust. This shadow, strangely enough, doesn't involve darkness but light. This was David's secret to not being afraid.

Back in the city, on our last evening, Kevin and I walk around the Plaza de Armas, an impressive government building constructed with white stones. Although Arequipa's name origin is "the place that lies behind the peak," Arequipa is not known as the city of shadow. Rather, because of the architecture, Arequipa is known as the "White City."[5] The white stones, called *sillar*, are the result of consolidated volcanic ash from the eruption thousands of year ago of a now-extinct volcano.[6] The walls of Arequipa and the breathtaking main square are fashioned from hewn volcanic rock. Peruvians took what exploded and built a city. A beautiful, white city. Nestled in the shadow of an awakening volcano, Arequipa is known not for darkness but for light.

I struggle with the shadow of cancer, but we all have our shadows, our places of darkness that try to creep in and become a friend. We all have our fears of change and loss, because if one bad thing can happen, why not a second? Or a third?

Maybe it is time to choose a different shadow, to rename a destiny, and take what was meant for destruction and carve out new stones and live. Maybe it's time to build a white city.

This I know: it is definitely time to step under the shadow of almighty God.

Sixteen

Not Half of Two

Arizona has always had its share of tall tales, thanks to the writing genius of authors like Zane Grey and Louis L'Amour, who painted Arizona with a rough and tumble mix of adventure and Old West idealism. Since those days, approximately four million of us have settled into the Phoenix metropolitan area, making it easy to believe we've become civilized as we drive our minivans to the mall before returning to our landscaped, air-conditioned houses. But you don't have to drive far to leave the city life behind and enter the land of scorpions, coyotes, and rattlesnakes.

On a sunny day, several years ago, my husband and I headed out to Weaver's Needle on the Peralta Trail to search not for the legendary gold that lies somewhere beneath the Needle's shadow but for a chance to photograph illusive wildlife.

At the trailhead, we met two guys loading equipment. Painted on the side of the truck were the words *Rattlesnake Control*. One man had an orange bucket and a long-handled grabber. The other carried the largest pair of tweezers I'd ever seen. We later learned it was used for picking up baby rattlers or for feeding live mice to caged snakes.

"Okay, I can't resist," Kevin said, walking over to the men. "Tell me your best rattlesnake story."

The older gentleman pondered for a few minutes and drawled, "Well, it involves the border patrol." He loaded the bucket back into the truck and turned to give us his full attention. "They pulled me over awhile back while I was driving in southern Arizona. I don't know if they were looking for drugs or illegals or what, but they motioned me out of the line. The back of my truck was full of fifty buckets of snakes."

He took a swig from his water bottle and spat on the ground. "I got out and said, 'There's rattlesnakes in there.'

"'Yeah, we've heard that one before,' they replied. One officer ignored my warning and reached for a bucket.

"I yelled, 'I'm serious! Don't touch that bucket!'

"He put his hand on his gun at his hip and pointed at me, 'Sir! Sit down over there and shut up!'

"So I did. The officer took the lid off a bucket with three Mojaves. One of the snakes extended its full length as it tried to escape. The border agent screamed like a girl. Yep, just like a little girl. You shoulda heard him."

The old snake catcher chuckled at the memory before delivering his punch line. "And then he wet himself. Yep, it's true." He smiled. "And that's my best story."[1]

We laughed in appreciation. Arizona tall tales never die.

"Did you get any rattlers today?" I asked.

He shook his head. "Nope. Too late in the day. They are already back in their holes."

We took off down the trail, heading for the Needle. Despite the old codger's opinion, we kept our eyes open for snakes. We covered ground quickly, hiking first along a creek bed and then ascending the switchbacks to the saddle. Weaver's Needle's one-thousand-foot spire rose impressively above us.

We attempted to get some photos of spiking century plants, the gold spires six to eight feet in the air. We skirted around one giant succulent—and its serrated two-foot-long blue-green leaves hanging over the trail—to avoid the pointed tips that can pierce to the bone.

Maneuvering around a century plant, we nearly missed him—a Gila monster sunning himself next to the trail, his eyes watchful. The Gila is the only venomous lizard in Arizona. He posed quietly while I snapped picture after picture, from a safe distance, of his orange-and-black-banded leathery skin, which is similar to Native American beadwork. The Gila was our first sighting of the lizard outside of captivity.

Like many desert creatures, the Gila is created to survive the harsh desert environment. Ninety-five percent of the lizard's time is spent below ground in its burrow. Some believe Gilas emerge only three to four times a year, eating large meals and storing fat in their thick tails.

The Gila monster spends most of its life alone.[2]

I understand the burrowing. The hiding. The seclusion.

I am tired of cancer. Tired of talking about it. Tired of writing about it. Tired of feeling like a prayer project. Tired of waiting for the other shoe to fall. Tired of opening social media and learning another friend has cancer. Tired of having cancer linked with my name. Tired of no longer being able to answer "Fine" when people ask a casual, "How are you doing?"

Will I ever be fine again?

The psalmist laments in Psalm 13:2, "How long must I wrestle with my thoughts and day after day have sorrow in my heart?" (NIV).

I am tired of the wrestling. I long to hole up in my grief and only come out for food.

The morning of my surgery, I awaken early. People have asked me if I'm ready and I reply in the affirmative. I joke about being able to put a huge check mark on my to-do list. I don't think I'm worried, but I didn't sleep well, having tossed and turned the entire night.

I gather loose socks and throw them into the laundry room. I put dirty dishes next to the sink. I grip my fingers around what I can control.

As a child, I remember Mom was always the last one to get in the car when we went on vacation. Dad would work his magic and pack the camping gear into every nook and cranny, plus the assorted belongings of four children. And food—canned goods, bread, and a cooler filled with bologna sandwiches.

We would climb into the station wagon with "the little girls," my two younger sisters, getting the middle seats, while my brother and I claimed the coveted window positions.

Then we would wait—wait for Mom. We chased mosquitoes out the open windows and declared war with siblings who dared to cross our inches of territory. We would wait, because Mom was mopping the floor.

With four young children and various pets with muddy paw prints, the only way Mom could guarantee a clean floor was to mop the linoleum while we were all seatbelted in a vehicle that was headed out of town. Mom wanted a clean floor when she returned home.

As a mom of four, I totally understand. After gathering the dishes, I head for the mop. My son walks out, ready to leave for an early class.

"I won't be here tonight," I remind him.

"Why?"

"Surgery today."

I see the child and the man on his countenance—the child who has forgotten and struggles to make a place for this view of his mom as a patient who needs care and the man who has experienced loss and knows too well what this could mean. I know I have displayed the same emotion on my face as I have grappled as a woman and a daughter with my mother's continuing cancer battle.

The child makes a joke about death, and rather than chastise him, I wrap my arm around his waist and remind him to take out the trash. I remember when he was fourteen and I was newly diagnosed. We were still stumbling around trying to grab words to talk to each other about what happened, because how do you talk about breast cancer with your mom when you are fourteen? How do you talk about cancer at any age?

At fourteen, he left a book on my pillow with a sticky note, penned in junior high scrawl, "You should read this book." The book, my son's frame of reference for cancer at the time, was a young adult novel about a boy with leukemia and the effects on his family. In the pages of that book, my son, the emerging man, provided me with a door opener to necessary conversations.[3]

"Maybe I can come home early," my son says as he grabs his textbooks.

I eye the stack of calculus and physics books under his arm. In a year of loss—when numbers came in doses of meds, rounds of chemo, and the cost of plane tickets—I envy him, having only to worry about the scholarly numbers on a page. Logging on to the family computer last week, I came across a document titled "Finding Mass of a Car." It took me a moment to realize the file was about math and not cancer.

Such is my life. His life. Our lives.

"Call or text your dad."

He nods. He turns back for one more quick hug. I squeeze the child and the man tight. I hear the door click shut. I can think to do only one thing.

I mop the floor.

Once again I find myself undressing and placing my belongings in a plastic bag before robing my bare skin in a "Property of the Hospital" gown. My husband knows the routine and asks for a heated blanket as I climb into the bed.

For the moment I am calm, unlike the week before when I faced the presurgery appointment. At that time anxiety blindsided me.

"What do you want me to do?" my husband asked as we sat together at the kitchen table. I had an appointment the following morning to go over the final details for my hysterectomy. My symptoms had continued to worsen.

Oh, the shadow—the lingering shadow of cancer.

"Routine," the surgeon had said, but since being diagnosed, I have learned *routine* never means take it for granted.

Cancer had not been kind that week. Mom had developed an infection. A friend's cancer had returned. And I now faced another surgery.

My husband knew all this.

"What do you need from me?" Kevin asked, the question quiet. He closed the morning newspaper on which he had been doing the crossword puzzle to give me his full attention.

I knew he was busy. I hated to ask him to come. When I had made the appointment I thought I was brave and strong.

But now?

I was fragile. Unraveling. Afraid.

He waited. His hazel eyes watched me.

Why couldn't I simply say the words? Why did the sounds stick in my throat? What pride or fear or warped internal image of strength kept me silent? Weren't we beyond this?

Two becoming one. It's not simply a physical oneness, but the peeling away of two lives learning to live together in union. The admitting of need.

It is more than sharing a home. A bed. A mortgage.

The Bible calls it a mystery. In the last few months, I have gathered clues by watching my parents. Somehow in our nakedness we let another see our wrinkles. Our faults. Our raw, stripped-down vulnerability.

Even after more than thirty years of marriage, a part of me still clings to independence. Singleness. Aloneness. Why do I avoid the union? The two becoming one?

I cleared my throat. "I need you," I said. My voice held the quavering of strength unhinging. "I need you to come with me."

"I'll make it happen," he said, getting out his planner. He erased appointments, changed his schedule.

"Thank you," I whispered.

"Of course." He glanced up, a quick smile on his face.

Of course. So simple. Why did I make it so difficult?

No longer half of two. Two becoming one.

Seventeen

When Anxious Thoughts Multiply

The doctor calls to report the surgery biopsy is negative. I do not have ovarian or endometrial cancer. A helium balloon of joy soars high with the news.

No cancer! No cancer! No cancer!

Before we can celebrate, the phone rings again. Mom has had a stroke. The joy balloon shrivels as it is yanked to earth by the tethered string.

After we learn more details, we realize Mom had the stroke two days earlier. After experiencing troubling symptoms, she told no one but continued with plans to work at a cranberry festival. When she started dropping things, friends took her to the hospital.

It is true, what they say, about apples not falling far from trees.

I am not recovered enough from surgery to get on a plane. Mom spends five days in the hospital and is released with no restrictions. Outwardly, she appears great. Then Mom, a woman who made her livelihood as a teacher with words, sends an email:

> Dear family J ak writing this ti see hie jajy errirs I jaie in ak e-mailo]
> I thiknk I shoiod maybe nit try to do thos today\ Love Gma

My sister Lisa makes the five-hour drive to check on Mom again. And worry comes to sit on my chest.

———

2:30 a.m. I swallow pain pills. I am not yet sleeping through the night since my surgery. I listen to my husband breathing. Watch the red clock numbers. 2:34. 2:37.

Will Mom be able to live alone? What other abilities has the stroke taken? Should she move in with one of my siblings? With me?

2:40. I am getting a lesson in math. Not in algebra or trig or calc, but all the way back to fourth grade, when Mom wrote my times tables on leftover recipe cards and I practiced them at the kitchen table. Multiplication.

Multiplication is essentially a shortcut to repeated addition. It is simpler to write 5×4 than $5 + 5 + 5 + 5$. This is true with numbers, but here during the night I discover multiplication can also be a shortcut to getting absolutely no sleep when applied to the thoughts going on in my brain.

Why is it that happy thoughts don't keep my eyelids from closing in the darkness? I could use a little pixie dust with Tinker Bell and Peter Pan, but no, I am left with anxious, worried thoughts that don't line up one by one to be added, but grow exponentially, taking over my brain. And my sleep.

"When my anxious thoughts multiply within me," the psalmist writes in Psalm 94:19. Apparently he also struggled with math.

The word *anxious* comes from a root word in Latin meaning "full of mental pain," "distressed," or "to strangle."[1] Tonight the last definition is true. Anxiety strangles thoughts of hope. Anxiety strangles peace. Anxiety strangles faith. Anxiety definitely strangles sleep.

What do you do when anxiety multiples within you and counting sheep doesn't cut it? (Obviously counting sheep is a simple addition problem, and I have advanced to higher math.) The psalmist writes, "When my anxious thoughts multiply within me, your consolations delight my soul" (Ps. 94:19).

Consolation is an old-fashioned word meaning "the act of consoling; comfort; solace."[2] When the psalmist struggled with anxiety, he would remember the goodness of God in the middle of the night. Rather than worry about what to wear to the next royal dinner or what his enemies were plotting, he focused on the helping, supporting, comforting side of God.

2:47. I swallow hard. Count out thanks.

Thank You that Mom seems to have no other lasting effects from the stroke. Thank You that she is getting excellent care. Thank You for my sister, who is able to check on Mom for all of us.

At first it is like counting sheep. The process is slow and forced, as I mentally shift my brain from negative to positive. The anxiety attempts to strangle me, sitting on my chest and squeezing out my breath. It is difficult to focus on anything resembling comfort. Where can I find relief? My mind went back to a hike I took shortly after Dad's death.

Night had left, but it was not quite dawn—the in-between of "still dark" and "not yet light." I found myself there, in the grieving. A cottontail bounded down a nearby wash, not with a hop but, rather, with his front feet and hindquarters coming together in a slight rocking motion. A mama quail darted across the trail in front of me, four babies toddling behind her in a straight line. *Ka kwah kah. Ka kwah kah.* Her black head plume bounced as she called to the slowest one, who raced behind her like a wobbling windup toy.

A young saguaro, three feet high, grew out of the stony ground in front of me. The cactus had pushed through a crevice in a boulder, splitting the rock in two. Years ago the rock served as a nursemaid, hiding the tiny black cactus seed. The shaded area had held in moisture and protected the seed from birds and other animals. The crack allowed rainwater to flow right to the growing saguaro and the rock had kept the water from evaporating in the desert heat. It had been the perfect hiding place until the saguaro was large enough to push skyward.

Drip. Drip. Drip.

Although the saguaro would eventually tower over the desert landscape, the plant grew slowly in infancy, reaching only one inch in the first eight years. The baby saguaro could not survive alone; it needed protection. The saguaro needed to grow in the hiding place of shadow.

I find myself needing that same shading presence, that same rock of hiding.

About the time Dad was diagnosed, I began memorizing large passages of the Bible with a group of women—a discipline I had tossed aside along with the charts of gold stars from Sunday school class. It all seemed a bit archaic to me.

Yet each week we would sit in a circle, women with ages spanning three generations, and open our Bibles. We memorized portions together—whole chunks of passages—because we knew living this loving, doing, walking life could drain the moisture right out of us. Like the tiny saguaro, we needed the water of His words flowing off our tongues, bathing our hearts. Verse by verse, drip by drip.

"Do not be anxious about anything, but in every situation, by prayer and petition, with thanksgiving, present your requests to God" (Phil. 4:6 NIV). We let the memorized truth-words drip down. In the desert, water runs to the lowest source, into cracks, into the tiny splintering places, and it is also true of our hearts. The moisture lands on waiting seeds, allowing plants to grow protected under the desert sun.

Philippians 4:6 contains twenty-one words, words that are easy to memorize but difficult to live out. Twenty-one words needed to rehydrate a life. Soaking words for people to actively drip into their relationships. Their spheres of influence.

Words for soul-gripping anxiety.

Women shared deep, the fissures where words from life had seeped out truth. Grandmothers, mothers, sisters, friends, we placed hands on shoulders and prayed for words to water seeds and grow tall in us.

I didn't know when I started the discipline that I would face soul-gripping anxiety at 2:30 a.m. I didn't know life was about to take huge pieces out of me and I would need His watering words to fill in the holes. I didn't know my view of God would be shaken and I would need to rediscover Him in His words of love written throughout the ages.

I didn't know that ten days after the stroke, Mom would have a heart attack. I board a plane. Despite my best efforts, anxiety climbs out of my suitcase and settles between my shoulders.

———

"Your mom kissed the face of Jesus twice in the past ten days," Mom's friend says as I rush to join my siblings in the ICU. "He sent her back."

Mom is pale but communicative, full of stories of her heart attack while she was driving and her helicopter ride for emergency surgery seventy miles away from home. She is happy one of the EMTs had Dad as a teacher. I wonder how learning about adverbs and prepositional phrases in ninth grade qualified this man to take care of her, but as is the way of small towns, there is comfort in the knowing and being known. I watch the swaying of her dangling turquoise earrings and can't help but notice her jewelry matches her hospital gown.

I struggle to wear matching earrings on my non-heart-attack days.

My siblings and I receive a crash course on new medical terminology. Ejection fraction. Hypercoagulability. Trousseau's syndrome. An endless parade of doctors order tests and keep us informed. A cardiologist. An oncologist. A hematologist. A social worker. An occupational therapist. A physical therapist.

The doctors come in a constant stream to talk to my siblings and me. The "Gathering of Suits," as we call them, soon turn their attention to Mom, as she asks about ischemic damage and thrombotic events and uses medical jargon from her years of training medical secretaries and transcriptionists, which included years of teaching college-level anatomy.

Our hearts warm as we see the mom we have always known and loved, although a bit pale and now sporting a stent, wearing her earrings and charming the doctors. The doctors anticipate several weeks of rehab and then she can go home. With Mom stable, we move out of the hotel across from the hospital and settle into the family acreage seventy miles away.

"Was this sign in the bathroom when we were here for Dad's funeral?" I ask my sister as she lugs suitcases into our childhood home.

She peers around the door frame to check out the white sign with red lettering taped to the mirror. "I don't think so."

Mom loves to hang inspirational sayings. She cuts them out and places them at strategic places throughout the house: on the hutch in the living room, on the bay window by the kitchen sink, and in the bathroom. I don't remember the sign being here four months ago.

I trace the red words with my finger—life blood written by a new widow adjusting to life without her husband of fifty-five years. *Do not be anxious about anything, but in every situation, by prayer and petition, with thanksgiving, present your requests to God*, the sign reads.

Did Mom also have her 2:30 a.m. watches of the night, where anxiety tried to steal sleep? In this, are the falling apples also close to the tree?

Can we gather water together for our heart cracks?

The grass crunches crisp under my feet as I step out into the new day, still dark in its infancy. I walk to the well on Mom's property.

"The chemicals need to sit overnight and then the water needs to run ten hours," Mom's friend said after he came and dumped gallons of bleach into the well. "Until it quits running black and the odor is gone."

Before her heart attack, Mom had a new hydrant put over the well, opening it to possible dirt and contaminants. The well needs cleansing before it is safe to drink.

I crank the lever full. I run a hose toward the neighboring field, where only short stubble remains from sentry corn stalks.

My siblings have returned to their families while I take my turn watching Mom, so I am all alone—a circumstance unknown to me. This is a home of family gatherings, my dad driving the Allis-Chalmers, grandkids playing with our childhood toys, and Mom rolling flour-covered memories with eager assistants in the kitchen.

The grain elevator to the north is awake, swallowing harvested fields into its belly, lights running day and night as farmers race against the clock. The smell of fall is in the air—combined with the strong smell of bleach from the hydrant, with black water running, the well pumping it down.

I have known the blackness. The darkness of fear as I boarded the plane after Mom's heart attack, racing the clock, wondering if it was Mom's harvesting time.

I didn't know when I sat with a circle of women back in Arizona and memorized Scripture that I would need to stand under the shelter of His Word, words I had hidden away in my heart. When I was stumbling around in the dark, I didn't have time to find a Bible or pull up thoughts on a computer screen or find an app on my phone. When I couldn't remember anything else about my faith, the verses I had memorized dripped into my soul cracks.

Even if it is not cancer, we all have words. Words from doctors. From family. From friends. From a boss. From a co-worker. From strangers. From those who are supposed to be closest to us yet who wound us the most.

The words absorb into skin, and the weight sinks down. The words sit, stir, and churn, like food poisoning of the soul, until 2:30 a.m. when you relive the words in "what if" nightmares.

Maybe you find yourself standing, like me, by a well, where the dirt of circumstances has putrefied your soul water and the blackness of night is all around you and you are all alone.

How do you run clean and free again?

At the well, I focus on the quiet, the darkness around me, and the fact that I am alone. In the absolute silence of a new day, as I stare into the star-filled sky, I hear the truth of Scripture I memorized in the past.

If the purpose of discipline is to prepare for what is to come, I know I am now standing in such a moment. The words find the smallest crevices, the deepest cracks, and penetrate down to the hardest places, washing away contaminants, watering seeds.

I stand on the property of my childhood home and once again gaze at the stars. Words I have memorized fill my mind—but not just words. The weight of the Word surrounds me. "The heavens are telling of the glory of God; and their expanse is declaring the work of His hands" (Ps. 19:1). Truth falls into place as my heart finds its home.

Somewhere during my journeying I began living an asterisk life. A life where Jesus is the name above all names, with one exception— at the bottom of the page, in fine print—Cancer. Cancer (with a capital C). Cancer had become the asterisk, the exception, the exemption, the deal breaker. I had let my circumstances define my faith. Cancer became magnified as God shrunk and the snake became a dragon. A loud, fire-breathing dragon.

"Keep the size of God in perspective," Chris Jackson and Dutch Sheets write in *Praying through Sorrows*. "He's the beginning and the end. If you judge Him only by the present circumstance, you will despair. The shortest moment of time is this present moment, but in grief the present moment seems to last for an eternity."[3]

Under night skies, I hear the star song and find perspective. God, who holds the universe in His hand, also holds me near His heart. This is mind-boggling. Lie shattering. Dragon stomping. Faith restoring.

I stand under the revealing knowledge of the stars, and in that moment love finds me. My breath blows white while Orion the Hunter shouts silent and the Big Dipper spills glory. I know what I have heard said is also true for me. We don't want an explanation of God; we want an encounter with Him. In an instant I know God surrounds me.

I stand without the noise of cousins and siblings and parents and family, with only the stars in the sky and the grain elevator belching corn dust, yet I sense Him. The One who loves me most. Jesus is with me by the well in the blackness. The silence completely fills. With Him.

I stumble out words.

Thank You for the doctor who took the time to sit on Mom's bed to hear her questions. I saw in his compassion that he understands our fear. I don't know what we would do without the lifeline of Mom's friends, who drive seventy miles each way to sit by her hospital bed. Thank You for my brother's steady wisdom when I called in a panic. I needed that. Help me . . . I don't know . . . just . . . help.

Be anxious for nothing. In everything . . . prayer. Be thankful. Make your requests known.

I did not realize until that moment that the discipline of finding beauty in the difficult and meditating on Scripture would allow the black to run out, the stench to pour free, and my soul water to be clean once again. Memorizing the Word of God multiplied the remembrance of His goodness and faithfulness. The discipline became a sheltering rock so seeds of life could grow. His Word subtracts soul-crushing anxiety.

Words in. Blackness, stench, and anxiety out.

I like that kind of math.

Eighteen

The Dance of Surrender

Music is the language of the soul. The sign hangs at the Musical Instrument Museum (MIM) in Scottsdale, Arizona. Room after room contains instruments from around the world. Drums. Lutes. Bells. Gongs.

The most interesting instruments, however, are not the traditional winds and brass, but what the docent calls "found instruments"—music makers created from objects that were originally intended for something else.

A pig bladder. A horse jawbone. A thistle. A gas can. A walrus stomach stretched as a drum.

The creativity of the instrument inventors amazes me as they took what was available in their everyday lives to fashion an instrument. Sometimes the playing of the song in the ordinary is the most challenging, as we struggle to find the tune.

Scrubbing the bathtub. At the bedside of a loved one. After a phone call from the doctor. The times when insides are taken out and stretched tight for all to see.

Could found music be the most beautiful song?

In Mom's bedroom, after several weeks of rehab, I notice her Autoharp, an instrument she hasn't played in years, along with some sheet music.

"I decided my life needed music again," Mom says when I ask her about it.

Mom has been practicing her found music. Songs strummed as a recent widow. Tunes sung as a patient whose cancer has spread to the lining of her abdomen. Melodies gritted out through the drumbeats of daily pain.

Mom has me send a family email that reads: "Thank you so much for your prayers. Last evening my devotional book had a great word for me: 'Trust Me and don't be afraid, for I am your Strength and Song. Do not let fear dissipate your energy. Instead, invest your energy in trusting Me and singing My Song.'[1] I went to bed singing!"

It is one choice to sing a song when life is happy. It is another to let others hear the most haunting melodies, set in a minor key. To compose night songs in prayer. "The LORD will command His lovingkindness in the daytime; and His song will be with me in the night, a prayer to the God of my life" (Ps. 42:8). I am humbled by the pure beauty of Mom's song.

As I sit on the corner of her bed, we talk about my kids and her grandchildren, about neighboring farmers as they harvest against the clock of an upcoming storm. She gives me detailed financial information. We chat about which flowers are still blooming, of how beautiful her peonies were this year.

And cancer. We talk about cancer. Mom is not sure she is ready to sing her last verse. The notes written inside her head tell her she will live at least as long as her parents before facing her *barra finale*, the end of her musical score. Still a decade shy of that inner timeline, she struggles to compose a new melody. Cancer has interrupted the story she has sung over her life, hijacking the tune. Arthur W. Frank writes that a serious illness is difficult because "the present is not what the past was supposed to lead up to, and the future is scarcely thinkable."[2]

I remember when I was a little girl going into my parents' room at night, unable to sleep because of a nightmare. Mom woke up, my presence in the room alerting her.

Mom told me to sing songs until I became tired. Or to pray. I climbed back under the covers in my own room and sang under my breath, whispering melodies into the shadows, not knowing four decades later I would still need to sing songs in the night when faced with life terrors.

Mom points me to music and prayer as we process her cancer—me as a daughter and she as a mom and both of us as women who love. I believe one of the greatest gifts we give our children is the willingness to talk about death and the eternal and to teach them to sing songs in the night.

"The LORD is the strength of my life; of whom will I be afraid?" (Ps. 27:1 ISV). Mom typed the verse in a family email when Dad was diagnosed. She hit send and the words traveled out into the atmosphere to four generations. She repeated the refrain at her own diagnosis and sings the words now as she recovers from her stroke and heart attack.

I am unsure how I misinterpreted the main chorus of my mother's life song, thinking I needed to do things in my own strength. I hum the notes, cautiously: "The LORD is the strength of my life."

"Dance as if no one is watching." I've seen this phrase on T-shirts, jewelry, and inspirational posters. The phrase encompasses the thought that a life should be lived with boldness. No fear. With abandon, expressing beauty and creativity. Even in night seasons.

It is a wonderful sentiment.

Unless you have two left feet.

I am a singer, not a dancer. The whole feet-brain-arms coordination is beyond my ability. Occasionally I go to a Zumba class at the fitness center and the phrase "dance as if no one is watching" comes back to taunt me. It's fine to have people watching you if you know what you are doing, but to know you are the center of attention because you are clueless is another matter. When everyone else goes right, I go left. When everyone is hopping, I'm stepping. Without fail, the instructor notices my clumsiness and comes to stand next to me, simplifying the steps. Slowing the movement. So I can get it.

I don't get it.

Finally, she laughs, throws up her hands in defeat, and returns to teaching the class. I am left to my own devices as everyone dances and steps around me.

Mark 14 tells the story of a woman who didn't get it either. Jesus is eating at the home of a Pharisee and a woman shows up with an expensive bottle of perfume, which she breaks and pours over Jesus. The woman kisses His feet, cries so hard she wets His feet with her tears, and then mops everything up with her hair. People are indignant, call her a sinner, and complain about the extravagant waste of valuable perfume.

She didn't get it.

She didn't get the fact that it is unacceptable to show up un-invited to an important person's home and then make a scene in front of the dinner guests. She didn't get the memo that warned against good people being touched by unclean sinners. She didn't get that there are proper ways to behave, and these ways do not include breaking open perfume bottles, crying all over somebody's feet, and using your hair as a towel.

She didn't get it.

Or maybe she did.

Hidden in the story is a sentence I have never seen before. When people complain, Jesus tells them to leave her alone. He says, "She has done what she could" (Mark 14:8).

She has done what she could. At first I read the phrase with a note of defeat. *Well, she has done what she could, the poor dear. Leave her alone.*

But then I examined the verses again.

She has done what she could. Not a cop-out statement. No. Absolutely, no. What she could do was costly. Over the top. Out of the box.

Beautiful.

She moved to the beat of found music and danced as if no one were watching. Extravagantly. Aroma floating throughout the entire room. The scent of the poured-out dance. A bowed-down, lips-to-the-feet, bending-low movement. Love unashamed.

The ones watching pointed fingers and were critical. Mean. Judgmental.

But Jesus said whenever the gospel is preached in the whole world, people will tell this woman's story. Why? Because of the beauty in her dance.

I imagine the people at the dinner party returned home and their families had some questions about why their garments smelled like perfume, because, well, beauty and love poured out clings to you. It gets on your clothes. It gets under your skin.

Those people who were at the party didn't return home to talk about the rubbery chicken or overcooked veggies or minimal decorations. They came home and said, "You'll never believe what happened tonight. There was this woman, and you should have seen her dance!"

Beautiful sacrifice. It must be talked about. It cannot be silenced.

My siblings and I decide Mom can't live alone any longer. When I ask Kevin what we should do, he says, "Nobody is going to be at peace until your mom is living with one of you. Someone needs to do it. Why not us?"

And so it is decided.

The last Sunday I am in Minnesota, Mom and I attend church together. Mom is not the only one who is welcomed with open arms. I have known some of these women since I was an awkward teenager, all pimples and long hair. They attended my wedding and several years later threw me a baby shower. They were the first people Mom called when I had cancer. Their lips have spoken my name in prayer.

The congregation sings the opening verse of an old hymn:

> All to Jesus I surrender
> All to Him I freely give
> I will ever love and trust him
> In his presence daily live.
>
> I surrender all. I surrender all.
> All to Thee, my blessed Savior, I surrender all.[3]

Mom leans into me. Close. "I need to go to the altar," she says. Mom walks—without her walker—to the front of the sanctuary. She stands, yielded and vulnerable before all.

Five friends surround her, decades-loved women who have walked this life journey, who have sung the night songs. They stand. Support. Pray. Pass Kleenex around.

I surrender all. Mom takes the first hesitant steps in this new dance.

A church leader bends double and weeps into his hands, not only for the challenge of my mom's circumstances, not simply for the saying good-bye to a lifelong friend, not merely for the closing of a chapter—but tears in the difficult beautiful, for the releasing of the fisted hands and the unfurling of the knotted tight. The *yes* in the abundant and the hearts opened wide in the lean. Jesus, hand extended, asks, "May I have this dance?"

This dance. This found music.

Away from a home of more than fifty years. Away from a familiar rhythm. Away to one bedroom after living in a three-story farmhouse. Away to the love of a daughter, but not the love of a spouse. Away for the singing of the final verse.

My mother, altar-bound, demonstrates the way.

I surrender all.

Nineteen

A Mystery Bigger
than the Unanswerable

Halfway between Tucson and Phoenix is a challenging hike that is especially beautiful during wildflower season—Picacho Peak. The mountain also has the rare distinction of being the site of the westernmost battle of the Civil War. A reenactment of the 1862 battle is done each year among the cactus.

Picacho Peak is an unusual geological formation, a mountain that bolts fifteen hundred feet above the Sonoran Desert floor, pitted and steep, like an unfinished sculpture, never smoothed or rubbed down. Right out of the parking lot, hikers are greeted with the following sign: *Travel at own risk. Trail beyond upper saddle is primitive. Not recommended for children under ten, inexperienced hikers, or dogs.*

What the sign says is true. Portions of the trail after the saddle are rugged, with chains drilled into the rock face to help hikers over the steeper sections. On a trek several years ago up the mountain, we hadn't hiked long before I realized I should have been more serious about my commitment to go to the gym. My heart pounded in my throat and I couldn't gasp enough air into my overworked lungs.

But as challenging as that hike was, it was nothing compared to a climb I ascended on that mountain almost two decades ago, a hike I made when my youngest was only six weeks old. I don't know what possessed me to think I could hike a mountain six weeks after having a baby, but I suppose it shouldn't have surprised me given my "I am strong, I am woman" mind-set. I wasn't foolish enough to think I could hike the entire peak and knew I couldn't take a baby on the steep sections that needed chains, but I figured hiking to the saddle wouldn't be difficult.

I was wrong.

I struggled up the trail and was soon the last one in the group. Another hiker, worried about me, loaned me his hiking stick so I wouldn't face-plant on the trail. Considering I was carrying the baby in a front pack, that was a wise precaution. Kevin put our two-year-old daughter on his shoulders and kept an eye on our older two kids as I wheezed my way past desert cactus and boulders. I felt every one of the extra pounds I had put on during my pregnancy.

I was oblivious to the cupped yellow-orange blooms of the Mexican poppy and the elongated clusters of blue lupines. I focused on one task—breathing.

Carrying yourself up a mountain is one thing. It's a completely different thing to carry another person. Even a very little person.

I sit in a circle of women, a group of ladies of all ages, and I ask, "What is something you are carrying that is too difficult for you?"

"My son's marriage."

"My grandchild's drug problem."

"My elderly parents."

"My husband's work schedule."

"My daughter's alcoholism."

Around the circle the answers come, from one woman. Then another. A total of eight women. Not one—not one mentions a personal struggle. Each woman mentions a family member. A child. A grandchild. A spouse. I mention my mother coming next week to live with us.

It is one thing to carry yourself up a mountain. It's another thing to carry another person.

———

My sister Lisa helps Mom pack in Minnesota, while I prepare a room for Mom in Arizona. My siblings and I decide to delay the sale of the farm until the spring, when the property will be covered in Mom's flowers. Perhaps, in reality, we cannot face the selling and the admitting of the ending.

Mom settles into our guest room, having packed a lifetime into four suitcases. She decides to continue with chemo, to fight for more time. We meet with a new oncologist and start a treatment schedule.

———

I watch the chemo drug drip like rainwater from the bag on the IV pole into a vein in Mom's arm. The clear liquid always surprises me; the lack of color masquerading as unassuming innocence. A closer inspection of the bag reveals these words: *Caution: Chemotherapy Drug. Handle with gloves. Dispose of properly.* Red biohazard bins sit in several corners of the chemo room.

"Why do you want more time?" someone asks Mom, soon after her move to Arizona, echoing a question in my own heart. Dad talked openly of heaven, but Mom would rather make a to-do list of goals to accomplish. As a former community college teacher for training medical secretaries, Mom is comfortable surrounded by doctors and hospitals, yet I can't help wondering, *Why is she holding so tightly to this life?*

"Because life is beautiful," Mom answers.

Stage-4-ovarian-cancer life is beautiful. Cancer-spread-to-the-lining-of-the-abdomen life is beautiful. Blood-clots-in-the-legs-and-lungs life is beautiful. Daily-blood-thinner-injections life is beautiful. New-widow-with-complicated-health-issues life is beautiful.

Family and friends come in a constant stream, with multiple generations around my table. We surround Mom with this beautiful life. Great-grandchildren play in the backyard or with trains on the carpeting, while Lisa's homemade cheesecake is served in the kitchen and dominoes are played in front of the television.

We take photos of Mom holding her children's children's children, an occasion we never dreamed would be possible two months earlier when Mom had her stroke and heart attack.

Answered prayer sometimes sits on a brown couch holding a new baby wearing a pink headband, while a two-year-old brother asks for another story. Sometimes a miracle clothes itself in a normal day. A beautiful, normal day.

I am surrounded by caring people, but the weight of overseeing Mom's care weighs on me. The learning curve to understanding the complexities of her medical condition is huge, giving me the opportunity to feel like a failure every day as we meet with her doctors. I am on a first-name basis with the pharmacist. Keeping track of Mom's list of medications is challenging, but the most difficult weight is watching her deal with pain. Some days we stay ahead and chase the pain, but too many days the pain chases us and eats at the edges of my sanity.

"What is overwhelming?" a friend asks one Sunday when I drag into church.

"Doctors assume I know the answers to questions about Mom's care that I don't even have a clue I should be asking," I say.

The backpack of my soul weighs me down. As we scale this new mountain, this mountain of pain, I can't imagine facing the death of my remaining parent. Too much. Too soon. The impending loss is crushing.

The pain only adds weight to the questions that have remained unanswered, lurking in the background since cancer came knocking on my family's door. The questions pile onto my shoulders, adding to the burden of the daily care and the thought of losing Mom.

What did Mom ever do to deserve this? Is there another medical avenue we should be pursuing? Why are some prayers answered and others are not? Does God have power? Is He good? What is the purpose of pain?

Some days I remember lessons learned under star-filled skies and sometimes the heavens are dark—and silent—with the only shouting being done inside my own head. My own heart. I trudge one more step up the mountain.

My heart echoes the words of C. S. Lewis: "Not that I am (I think) in much danger of ceasing to believe in God. The real danger is of coming to believe such dreadful things about Him. The conclusion I dread is not 'So there's no God after all,' but 'So this is what God's really like. Deceive yourself no longer.'"[1]

I know it is the grief talking, but I can't stop the questions. I have been on this faith journey long enough to know in all relationships there are seasons of closeness and seasons of distance. And you don't abandon the whole thing when you are groping around in the darkness, trying to figure it out, but I am weary of the journey.

In the book *Praying through Sorrows*, the authors Dutch Sheets and Chris Jackson write, "Between the promise of recovery and the completed miracle lies a vast graveyard of Christian faith, and, for at least a portion of their lifetimes, the majority of Christendom lives there. Waiting for breakthrough, believing for the promises, and looking to the appointed hope, they struggle to stay the course."[2] I can relate. I want answers. Sometimes there are none.

John Wessells, who ministers to people with brain injuries, writes about the tension of unanswered questions: "Because to us, the only way the situation can ever make sense is if they can be whole again. Healed. The truth is, we think *answers* are the only way we'll ever feel better about the messiness of our circumstance. The mystery of it. The *unanswerableness* of it. Only an answer—a visible, knowable purpose—will take away the pain."[3]

Would someone please hand me the remote control so I can change the channel? I am weary of reality shows. Can't we watch *Wheel of Fortune* instead and spin for another chance to solve the puzzle and win some money? Can't I buy another vowel? Unfortunately, I keep landing on "lose a turn."

Well-meaning people want to join in our game. They want to take their spin at the wheel. The unanswerableness of pain and loss makes everyone uncomfortable, so in an effort to fill in the awkwardness, people give advice. Too much advice. If their great-aunt Matilda had cancer, they know all the answers for each and every type of cancer.

Solutions. Dietary changes. Exercise regimes. Prayer schemes.

"Choose the letter g, and then you will have the answer!" Armchair contestants. People fight for the remote in an effort to maintain control or argue for a chance to spin the wheel again. Some days I want to throw it all at them and say, "If you think you have the answer, you be in charge for a while!" The wheel lands on "bankrupt."

I am tired.

Tired.

Tired.

And heart sick.

I *hate* what cancer is doing to my mother.

Mom is the one who picks up the remote. She lowers the volume. "When your dad was diagnosed with cancer and he was in surgery, I focused and prayed on Psalm 131," she tells me quietly, her face pinched, waiting for the pain meds to kick in.

I had forgotten the details of the psalm in the deafening roar of pain, the ear-splitting howl of the unanswerable. I pick up my Bible and thumb to the correct place.

"O Lord, my heart is not proud, nor my eyes haughty; nor do I involve myself in great matters, or in things too difficult for me. Surely I have composed and quieted my soul; like a weaned child rests against his mother, my soul is like a weaned child within me. O Israel, hope in the LORD from this time forth and forever" (Ps. 131:1–3).

The paradox is not lost to me. Mom is content to be the child, and she is asking me to stop trying to be in control. Stop trying to be the parent. Stop trying to understand the incomprehensible and instead be content to rest and let God be in charge. I have gone searching for answers from wise theologians like C. S. Lewis, but Mom speaks the words, through the psalms, that allow me to unload a few bricks out of my soul's backpack.

I inspect my Bible again. Psalm 131 is a psalm of ascents, a song sung by the pilgrims as they traveled into Jerusalem, a song sung to take their minds off their journey as they climbed in elevation. A song my mother encourages me to sing as I climb this mountain.

"I do not involve myself in things too difficult for me." I falter the words. Hesitate toward the strength of a God bigger than the unanswerable. Attempt to embrace this mystery.

"I am like a child who rests against his mother," my mom whispers.

"Hope in the Lord," we sing in two-part harmony. We travel together up the mountain.

Twenty

The Most Brave

As winter continues in the desert, we wait for the rains that come this time of year, the quiet, soaking storms that have none of the bravado and rage of the summer monsoons. The moisture of winter rains soaks into the desert, preparing the soil for wildflowers to bloom. For me, spring begins with the arrival of the poppy and ends with the blooming of the giant saguaro, an event that draws the white-winged doves to the top of the cactus. I still remember the first year I noticed the saguaros' flowers as a younger desert dweller.

Sunrise was seventeen minutes away. I increased my pace, wanting to reach a clearing. A cactus wren sang the morning song on a towering saguaro, the cactus heavy with arms in the grayness. After a few notes, the bird fluttered upward, seeking comfortable footing among the spines.

I reached a large, flat rock in the midst of a saguaro forest. The spot reminded me of a miniature Pride Rock from *Lion King*, but instead of lifting the lion cub, Simba, I raised my camera toward Four Peaks, the distant mountains, waiting for the golden arrival. Birds ceased their antiphonal singing as they rested silent, waiting with me for the first brush of color on the horizon. We reached the fermata, a hold on the musical score, and paused in anticipation.

The conductor raised his baton to the symphony of a new day. The silhouettes of mountains appeared first, followed by outlines of bushes and cactus. Pale yellow turned to tangerine. The light revealed what I had not seen. On the crown of each saguaro, a white-winged dove sat, perched among the wreath of three-inch, creamy-white flowers. Each bloom had opened the night before and had only a few hours to be pollinated. The scent of the flowers, like ripe melons, lured in the doves and other birds during the day and long-tongued bats in the evening for a one-day convention at the cactus hotel.[1]

Each saguaro blossom has only twenty-four hours to bloom in glorious splendor. Only twenty-four hours to guarantee the expansion of future generations of towering giants. Only twenty-four hours.

I lifted my camera to document what life looks like when you only have one day. The doves drank nectar and joined again in the song.

Winter rains delay and the desert waits to bloom. I tuck underwear next to two pairs of black pants and roll up four colorful scarves—two teal and two purple—that coordinate with every outfit. The scarves surround twelve days' worth of seventeen different prescriptions: Pravachol, Protonix, Cozaar, Xeralto, Oxycontin. A week ago when the fever hit, when tests were run at the doctor's office and I woke at midnight and 4:00 a.m. to administer medication, I did not believe this day would come. I did not think I would be packing two suitcases for my mom to spend Christmas with my brother.

Even as I throw in a hot water bottle and a bottle of Miralax, I wonder at the sanity of such a plan—to send my mother on a plane with her health issues. How much easier it would be to stay here.

Yet isn't this our role as women who love—the going and the letting go, the continual severing of the umbilical cord? I didn't realize until today that it works both ways.

When I was eighteen, I walked into the house and declared to my parents that I wasn't going to college after all. Instead, I was going to move to northern Canada and live among the Cree and Ojibwe in a small cabin with wood heat and no running water. I thought I was brave and adventurous.

It was years later before I realized the most brave person that day was my mother—who packed up her own dreams for my life as she stood in my pink bedroom, folding my jeans next to my long underwear and tucking in wool socks next to the down vest she had purchased for me—a living example that dreams are not always sensible and destiny does not always equate to safety.

And love, love is about letting go.

Mom boards a plane to spend Christmas with my brother. It is not sensible or safe with her health conditions, but I drive her to the airport and do what she has always done for me—give her dream wings.

Her courage amazes me as she packs up her fears about her health and worries about if she can make it to the bathroom in time and crosses the continent to be near her son. Again, she is the most brave.

Sometimes bravery wears sensible black shoes and tucks an extra Depends in her purse. Sometimes bravery trusts your safety, and the safety of those you love, to God.

———

How do you live when you have a diagnosis of limited days? What do you say when the doctor is unsure if the cancer or the blood clots will kill you? How do you pray when doctors talk of life-extending options, not disease-healing alternatives? What if these questions aren't hypothetical but involve someone you love?

I flip the calendar to another year. Friends and acquaintances are making goals and resolutions filled with hope, but I can't help but reflect on last year and wonder how I ever survived. I consider the future and fear I face more of the same—a difficult and soul-wrenching continuation of days.

I struggle to hold on to the lessons taught in Psalm 131, to be a child who leans and rests and does not strive after things too difficult. But this is my mom, and I want more. As a person of faith who believes God promises good things to those who love Him, I sometimes can't help thinking, *If this is how you treat your friends, I sure wouldn't want to be your enemy.*

Do I even want to write that here for everyone to read? Do I want others to know my deepest secrets, whispered in the pain and darkness during the watches of the night?

Is this you?

It is me. Sometimes.

Just as it is sometimes you and it is sometimes not you. Sometimes you have faith, hope, joy, and gratitude, and life is good and you can't wait for your feet to hit the ground running into a new day. But lately life has been hard. You know if you focus on what you have lost, and might possibly lose in the days ahead, you will go insane. You will spiral into a really, really bad, stinking, dark place.

After the day Mom pointed me to Psalm 131, I penned these words in my journal as my goal for this season: *Enjoy the one moment. The gift of one.* I might not have more, but I have this one.

One sunrise. One memory. One kiss. One squeezing of the fingers. One prayer. One conversation. One reason to be thankful. One "it was evening and it was morning." One day.

The gift of one keeps me going.

I want to be present in the difficult beautiful of this found music, to walk this journey with my family, my friends, and my God. And to know, even in this desert season, there is time to focus on what is essential. Roy Lessin, poet and author, says, "There is always time enough in a day to do God's will."[2] Enough time, even in the midst of terminal illness. Enough time, even on the ending of days.

I must choose, with God's help, to enjoy the gift of Mom's life, as it is lived in a series of moments in a twenty-four-hour day.

But how do I pray for the dying? Mom dying? The challenge I find as a person of faith is I still want to see her healed. I want to see her whole. I continually struggle with a side to my belief system that demands this as the only tenable solution, even though death is part of this life.

Are prayer words even possible?

I believe God has created each one of us for specific purposes. Good purposes. Ephesians 2:10 says, "We are His workmanship, created in Christ Jesus for good works, which God prepared beforehand so that we should walk in them."

Acts 13:36 states, "Now when David had served God's purpose in his own generation, he fell asleep" (NIV). King David fulfilled God's purposes, first as a shepherd tending his father's flocks and later as a king. He wrote many of the psalms, providing words that touched not only his generation but every generation following. He died—fulfilling God's purpose.

Even Jesus talked about completing an earthly assignment. While praying to His Father, Jesus said, "I have brought you glory on earth by finishing the work you gave me to do" (John 17:4 NIV).

Finished work that glorifies God. These words guide my prayers. I pray Mom will fulfill all the purposes of God for which she was created on this earth. It's the prayer I prayed for my husband's parents when they had cancer. It's a prayer I prayed over my dad.

I tuck her into bed in the same bedroom I once tucked in our girls. Instead of stuffed animals, a penguin collection, and Polly Pockets, the room now contains a smiling photo of my dad sporting a Mickey Mouse tie, pictures of other family members, a worn Bible, and a notepad for Mom to scribble lists. I check the oxygen machine. I hand Mom her nighttime meds. I position her water bottle and cell phone—in case she needs to reach me in the middle of the night. I turn on a worship CD to play quietly in the background. Sometimes I read from a devotional. And sometimes the in-between life encroaches—the laundry, the dirty dishes, the phone calls—and it's a rush and a blur.

But other times, as I turn out the light, I pray she will live each twenty-four hours to the fullest as she moves toward the fulfillment of God's purposes for her life.

While Mom lives out these purposes, we continue to wait for desert rains. We wait for the first arrival of desert poppies to the final hurrah of the twenty-four-hour saguaro blossoms. While the poppy arrives to full desert sun, the flowers of the saguaro stage the final anthem of springtime in the darkness, attracting bats and other nighttime creatures before crescendoing into the sunlight for the final blooming.

According to Frederick Turner, "Standing sentinel in the forbidding desert wastes, the saguaro constitutes a grand, green answer to our oldest questions, 'What are Life's chances against Death?'"[3]

What are life's chances against death? The desert flowers hold the promise of an answer beyond the waiting, to a hope I will one day see.

This. Yes, this, I believe.

I believe this for my mom, who has lived the cycle of nearly seventy-eight years, who stands in the heat of full desert sun and struggles to breathe in desert darkness, who is so tired, so very tired in the waiting. I pray her one-day blooms continue to attract others to her heaven-stretched arms as she brings glory to God while she fulfills her God-given destiny.

And my heart pleads. One more. One more.

Twenty-one
Finding God in Community

Dawn is close, so I leave the flashlight in the car. While Kevin is home with Mom, I have come early to the Desert Classic Trail, with only Venus, the morning star, still shimmering in the sky, not yet giving way to the sun. The air is clean, the desert having heaved a sigh of relief from the winter rains last evening. The water has washed the color from the atmosphere, allowing only the palest of pink to tint the sky, like too much water on a watercolor painting.

I pass a staghorn cholla and an adolescent saguaro, waiting to turn fifty years old so it can earn its first arm. A dry brittlebush and several creosote bushes guard my destination, an outcropping of boulders where the petroglyphs are located. The rocks are covered in geometric shapes: spirals, circles, and swirls, along with drawings of humans and bighorn sheep. I place my palm above one of the spirals, not touching the ancient drawings. My stretched fingers span the circumference.

I can't help but wonder who sketched these rock pictures years ago. Were the creators of the petroglyphs the graffiti writers of their day? Was it considered vandalism to inscribe an image on a rock face? Or were they considered great artists of the culture?

Were they compelled by the need to imprint the proof of their existence on what was then the most permanent object available? A sense of "we came, we lived among these boulders, and we will not be forgotten"?

Do we also have the need?

Several years ago on a trip to Flagstaff in northern Arizona, Kevin and I stopped at a picturesque roadside church: Chapel of the Holy Dove, a primitive wedding venue with breathtaking views of the nearby mountain that are visible from the floor-to-ceiling windows in the A-frame structure. The beauty was marred by graffiti throughout the entire building—on the walls, on the benches, on the lectern, and even on the stone altar.

Written in black marker: "Josh and Steph engaged. 6/17/2010." Scrawled in red ink: "Hi Lew. From Adam." Countless names and signatures of those who had stopped in this tiny place were inscribed in the wood beams.

And prayers. "Thank you God for your healing and blessing. Bless my sons. Thank you God for the money to go on our dream trip." After the prayers were signatures: "Debbie, Dave and Gordon."

What need do we have to inscribe our name to a place and declare, "I was here!"? Do we each contemplate ways to leave a legacy, something that will outlive us? Something that will serve as a witness to our existence?

In the movie *Shall We Dance?*, actress Susan Sarandon talks about this need. "We need a witness to our lives. There are a billion people on the planet. What does any one life really mean? But in a marriage, you're promising to care about everything. The good things, the bad things, the terrible things, the mundane things. All of it. All the time. Every day. You're saying 'Your life will not go unnoticed because I will notice it. Your life will not go unwitnessed because I will be your witness.'"[1]

The movie is referring to marriage, but I believe this need for a witness also pertains to friendship and community. There is a

Spanish proverb that states, "Life without a friend is death without a witness."[2] I was surprised my parents gave me *carte blanche* to write about their cancer stories. "You don't need to run anything by us first," they said, giving me permission to blog about their struggles.

Eventually I realized they wanted me to record their story, to give words to their suffering. To inscribe their names into paper and declare, "We were here."

One of the greatest gifts we give those who are suffering is to stand with them and announce, "I will be your witness." Humans have a basic need for companionship. For friendship. Everything about our bodies was created for touch, for closeness.

Our skin, alone, tells us this.

Skin is amazing. Averaging a mere nine pounds, the skin is more than a visible package we use to display ourselves to the world, holding the shape of our bodies in place and keeping our internal organs from spilling out.

"The skin doesn't exist merely to give the body an appearance. It is also a vital, humming source of ceaseless information about our environment,"[3] writes Dr. Paul Brand, who was a renowned hand surgeon and leprosy specialist until his death in 2003. Our skin reacts to wind, temperature, humidity, and light. It is the first line of defense against disease. "Skin is tough enough to withstand the rigorous pounding of jogging on asphalt, yet sensitive enough to have bare toes tickled by a light breeze."[4]

Through our skin, we experience the softness of a baby's cheek, the silkiness of a flower petal, the stiffness of a new pair of jeans, and the splash of ocean waves. We are not covered with feathers or scales or fur. We are covered with skin. "More than any other species, our skin is designed not so much for appearance as for relating, for being touched."[5]

Humans—created with so much skin—were meant to be touched. We see this in the truth of God coming to earth as a baby, entering this world with skin, becoming Emmanuel, God with us. *With us*:

in the scratchy hay in the manger and soft swaddling of strips of cloth in the hands of his mother, the warm breath of Joseph on his face. *With us*: with feeling and touch and pain and fatigue. *With us*: wearing skin.

Now it is our turn—to love with skin. To be "God with us" to others. But what do we do when we encounter the intense pain of a hurting world, when we are forced to face the unimaginable?

Our tendency is to pull back, to step away, to avoid pain and suffering, or to become numb. But the essence of our faith asks us to do the opposite, because love with skin steps forward—even closer. Skin was meant to be touched, and skin that is numb isn't healthy.

We, who love with skin, must move closer into the breathing, groaning, writhing mess of this world. In doing so, we explain God. When Jesus came to earth as a living, breathing, skin-covered person, He became the walking-around example of God. According to John 1:18, "He has explained [God]."

This God—who is all mysterious and wondrous, who is beyond comprehension and imagination, who can't be gazed on with the human eye because of His blinding glory and power—Jesus explained Him. Not so much with words, but with actions. By moving among people in their hurt. By touching people in their pain. By peering into the deepest places of their spiritual need. And by loving them.

He didn't only make eye contact. He made skin contact.

As followers of Jesus, you and I are containers of God. We are containers of the living God! We get to explain God.

As Kay Warren writes in *Dangerous Surrender*, "This is our prime task . . . to make the invisible God visible to a world that doesn't yet recognize him. We have the opportunity to be with another person in their need, thus 'explaining' God."[6]

In this season, I need community more than ever. In this bare-bones landscape, where giant oak trees and overflowing gardens have been removed and it is all spine and thorn and barrenness. As the pain seeks to isolate me and streamline our lives to the basic essentials, I need friends to be my witnesses—witnesses not only to my life but for God when I forget. I need others to be God with skin.

In a week marked with chemo and the worst day yet in this struggle with pain, I watch my mom attempt to hide it from me, but some pain cannot be masked no matter how hard we try. Hearing moans escape from the depths of her being, I can't help but wonder, along with the wise men in the Christmas story, "Where is He?" (Matt. 2:2).

After long travels from far-off places, the wise men arrived in Jerusalem with one pressing question: "Where is He?" Where is the purpose of our quest? Where is the destination of our journey? Where is the one we have heard about?

If the wise men were considered wise because they came seeking answers, then are we also wise when we ask questions in our journeys of darkness seeking the light?

All I know is I don't feel wise. Helpless would be a more accurate term.

"Where is He?"

In the pain. In the suffering. In the agony. Where is He?

I have participated in arguments in the past about the goodness of God, the purpose of pain, and the evils of a fallen world, but theology pales when it is much more than theory and it is your mom who is suffering. *My* mom.

"Where is He?"

In the book *The Problem of Pain*, C. S. Lewis prefaces, "I was never fool enough to suppose myself qualified, nor have I anything to offer my readers except my conviction that when pain is to be borne, a little courage helps more than much knowledge, a little human sympathy more than much courage, and the least tincture of the love of God more than all."[7]

Tincture. A tint. A slight trace. The smallest bit.

When painting a room, the smallest amount of tint can make a difference to a gallon of pure white paint. Drops of yellow, orange, or red will provide a warm, inviting, and homey tint. Drops of blue, green, or purple will create a refreshing and cool tint.

In matters of pain, sometimes all we need is the smallest evidence of the love of God to tint our perspective.

"Where is He?"

———

On Mom's seventy-eighth birthday, we go out for a birthday breakfast. We return home to queasiness, exhaustion, and more pain. Mom spends the late morning and afternoon resting. I am unsure if she will have energy for the planned evening activities, but she declares herself ready to go when 6:00 p.m. rolls around. We drive downtown, maneuvering our way through masses of people to find our reserved spot in the parking garage near city hall, where Kevin meets us. We walk a few blocks to our destination—an old fire truck, the fifth entry in the Festival of Lights parade.

We settle Mom next to the driver and find our places in the back of the truck, next to other city officials and their families. It is Mom's first ride in a parade since she was a candidate for homecoming queen in high school. She smiles and waves her beauty queen wave to the gathered throng.

This alone would have been a special birthday memory.

But my husband has a surprise in place. Earlier, Kevin walked up and down the street and whispered a secret plan to those claiming turf along the parade route.

In the fire truck, we follow a dancing group decked out in purple with white lights and their music blaring "Let It Snow." As our fire truck rolls down the street, a lady watching the parade from a folding chair, off to the right, bundled in blankets, yells out above the music, "Happy birthday, Lois!"

Mom turns in surprise.

"How did she know it was my birthday?" Mom asks the driver. He smiles, a conspirator in the secret.

A few feet later a man holding a toddler shouts, "Happy birthday, Lois!"

Mom smiles and waves back.

"Happy birthday, Lois! Happy birthday, Lois!"

All along the parade route Mom hears the words. Strangers, who agreed to participate in a birthday surprise, call out greetings to a woman they have never met, shining like stars on a difficult day. In a difficult season. In a difficult year.

"Friends have the power to reintroduce us to God," authors Dutch Sheets and Chris Jackson write.[8] My husband is that friend on this day, as he orchestrated others to participate in the reintroducing.

In their smiles, in their shouts, in their mittened waves, I see more than a little human sympathy. I discover more than a tincture of God's love.

I experience the answer to the gallon-sized question "Where is He?"

Here on the back of a 1936 fire truck, in a parade aptly named the Festival of Lights, I know the answer.

He is right here. Wearing skin.

Twenty-two
The Bully in the Mirror

The morning of my birthday—a Sunday—starts slow and difficult. Mom suffered a sleepless night due to the steroids needed to prep her body for chemo. We fiddled with oxygen levels several times and Mom tried moving to a chair, but nothing brought restful slumber.

"Let's stay home from church today," I suggest, minutes before we need to leave. Mom just finished breakfast and is still in her jammies.

"What?" Mom exclaims. "We are going to church! I won't wear my compression stockings. They take too long to put on. I'll wear my pajama pants and my slippers."

And off we go.

Mom is greeted by many people in her comfortable chair in the back of the sanctuary. She might model pajama pants and slippers, but she also wears a stylish blouse, earrings, lipstick, and a necklace she made with my sister Renae the week before. It's a birthstone charm necklace—one bead for each of the thirty-two members of her immediate family—kids, spouses, grandkids, and five great-grandchildren. She fingers the beads and mentions each person's name when anyone compliments her jewelry.

I can't escape the thought of a queen holding court. When the singing starts, I don't join in. I sit back and watch Mom in her pink fuzzy slippers, eyes closed, focusing on her Jesus. Some gifts come without wrapping paper.

At our last oncologist visit, Mom had a list of "what if" questions for the doctor as we detailed breathing problems, blood pressure issues, swollen legs, and blood clots. Mom, the multitasker, even in illness. Finally, her oncologist stopped her with a touch to her arm.

"Live your life, Lois. Live your life."

Today she demonstrates how to fully live that life. In the face of her own monumental health issues, she offers me an unexpected gift. The reason Mom insisted we attend becomes clear when the church members surprise me with cake, a basket of cards, and a secretly organized singing of "Happy Birthday" when I stand before the congregation to make an announcement. I am embraced by community.

Ever since I was a little girl, Mom made certain my birthdays, and the birthdays of my siblings, were special. Sometimes we had parties with friends, but each year we had the opportunity to choose the evening meal and pick out a cake for Mom to make: a train, a bear, a guitar, or even a banana-shaped cake that morphed into a yellow slug. Mom created each one. In later years, for her grandchildren, Mom (and Dad) always called to sing "Happy Birthday," mailed a card with money enclosed, and sent a family email asking Jesus to bless the birthday person in the year ahead.

After the busy morning, followed by lunch with family under the cat's claw vine in our backyard, I figure we will cancel our evening plans. Again, Mom will have none of that talk as she resumes the role of parent orchestrating a birthday for her little girl.

We load up people, a wheelchair, multiple cameras, and Mom's oxygen tanks, and head to the Desert Botanical Garden for the Chihuly glass display, a traveling exhibit of impressive glass sculptures amidst the desert landscape. We go at 4:00 p.m. so we can catch the light on the sculptures before and after the sunset.

In the garden, we catch our breath at the beauty. Blue ribbons of glass shoot up from an organ pipe cactus. A Medusa fireball of orange and red glass bursts in an explosion of color among towering saguaro giants. A forest of green-and-red-thorned glass spikes shares ground with the paloverdes.

The beauty of the light and glass is emphasized in the sparseness of the desert landscape. Each flowering red chuparosa bush, each prickly pear cactus, each wild lavender stem has plenty of space to stand out bold and beautiful against the endless dirt and scattered boulders. Unlike a Midwestern garden overflowing with dahlias, peonies, lilies, and a riotous display of blooms, the beauty of a desert garden is in the eye of the beholder, as the glass sculptures and desert plants are framed in barrenness.

Author and former park ranger Edward Abbey writes, "It has been said, and truly, that everything in the desert either stings, stabs, stinks, or sticks. You will find the flora here as venomous, hooked, barbed, thorny, prickly, needled, saw-toothed, hairy, stickered, mean, bitter, sharp, wiry, and fierce as the animals. Something about the desert inclines all living things to harshness and acerbity."[1]

Our son has an up-close-and-personal encounter with one of those stickered, mean plants while backing up to achieve good lighting for a perfect photo. Prickly pear cactus thorns pierce the pocket of his jeans, forcing him to take a trip to the restroom to remove them.

The apostle Paul once begged God to remove a thorn from his flesh,[2] and as a desert dweller, I understand the importance of not allowing a thorn to remain, whether a small barb embedded in the pad of Mollie's paw or a three-inch devil's claw that grips the entire toe of a hiking boot. Thorns not removed only prick and fester.

I have done my own begging in regard to the thorn of cancer. I am still in the process of learning what Paul found to be true: even when the thorn remains, there is grace. Sufficient grace. And Christ's strength for weak places.

Thorns are borne so much easier when pulled free with a twist and a yank, even if a spot of blood remains. I prefer dealing with thorns in this way, yet living daily with the pricking and the festering remains our difficult reality.

At the Desert Botanical Garden, our group of ten snaps photos on six cameras as we attempt to capture light and record memories of the beautiful against a sparse week of the difficult. After photographing desert plants, the cameras swing to document people.

Pink fuzzy slippers. A green and silver oxygen tank. Grown-ups posing like desert animals. Laughter. Photobombing. A visiting nephew/cousin joining the silliness. Hands held. Real smiles. Sunset peeking behind silhouettes.

For a couple of hours, we are a family in a garden. A mom. A grandma. A daughter. A grandchild. A husband.

Normal people.

For a couple of hours, time slows down. No talk of cancer. No talk of time running out. No talk of terminal. Numbers became silent as we live in the moment.

We discover much more than glass sculptures as we zoom in and focus close. We discover sufficient grace for the thorn.

Kevin's back strains as he pushes Mom around one last loop of sculptures as we attempt to lengthen the memory of this trip and delay the car ride back to reality. One glance at Mom, and I know she is tired. The scarf around her neck is dangling to one side. Her cheeks are flushed with color, but the lipstick on Mom's mouth has worn off. She has not reapplied it.

This, more than anything, tells me how she is doing.

I never knew my mom was fanatical about her lipstick. I never knew.

Since elementary school my friends have complimented me on my classy mother. She always dressed for town and wouldn't have imagined in a million years going to the hardware store in her paint clothes to purchase an extra gallon. She would change first. And apply her lipstick.

Perhaps the habit was a throwback from the years her family went to town during the Depression, once a week, dressed in their Sunday best. It was an event. Farm chores were left behind for a few short hours while the family replenished supplies in Clark, South Dakota, four miles away.

Mom never taught me how to apply lipstick. I was an avowed tomboy, and Mom must have despaired of ever training me to be a lady. Yet she performed her appropriate motherly duties, teaching me the proper etiquette about wearing clean underwear in case I was ever in an accident.

I never realized her love affair with lipstick until I was at St. Mary's Hospital in Rochester after her heart attack. My sister and I tried to take her for a walk down the hall and she wouldn't go until she had put on her lipstick. She shuffled between the nurse and my sister in her slippers and ratty blue hospital gown, her lips painted dark pink.

I didn't realize it until three months later when she was living in Arizona and was back in the hospital. I told her, "Mom, you don't need your purse. I'm bringing it home." Mom said, "Just give me my lipstick." Or until the time last week when the nausea from chemo was so bad we headed for the ER in the evening. I grabbed the laptop, the insurance cards, water, and a blanket. When we arrived in the waiting room, I noticed Mom brought only one thing—gripped in the palm of her hand—her tube of lipstick.

The Broadway musical *Annie* declares you are never fully dressed without a smile. My mother would agree with that statement, provided that smile was sporting the latest shade of red.

Mom comes from a generation when lipstick was a symbol of femininity, when Mrs. Cleaver greeted her husband with a kiss at the door while wearing a dress and pearls, balanced on high heels, her lipstick neatly in place.

But it is more than that.

The British soldier Lieutenant Colonel Mercin Willet Gonin, an eyewitness to the German Bergen-Belsen concentration camp, recounted a story shortly after the camp's liberation when a box arrived.[3] The needs were so desperate. Eager hands ripped open the box only to find it contained lipstick. Lipstick! What idiot possibly thought a tube of lipstick could heal the atrocities done by the Nazis?

Turns out the idiot was a genius.

The Nazis had stripped the women of their dignity. Of their families. Of their belongings. Of their identities. They had tattooed a number on their arms and said, "You are nothing. Nobody." Night after night. Day after day. The message had been pounded into these women's heads. Into their hearts.

But the lipstick whispered a different story.

The British soldier reported, "Women lay in bed with no sheets and no nightie but with scarlet red lips, you saw them wandering about with nothing but a blanket over their shoulders, but with scarlet red lips. I saw a woman dead on the postmortem table and clutched in her hand was a piece of lipstick."[4]

In a world that had stripped them down and left them bare, the lipstick whispered, "You are somebody. You are a woman. And you are beautiful."

Maybe Mom's fascination with lipstick isn't so strange after all. If a woman in a concentration camp can rediscover her beauty, why not a cancer patient?

I remember my own struggles with beauty after my diagnosis.

Sometimes cancer is a terrorist, exploding like a bomb in your life, causing mayhem and destruction. Other times, cancer is a bully, making daily demands for your lunch money. It was the lunch money losses that caught me off guard, surprising me with their difficulty. For me, one of the hardest things was going bra shopping after my surgery. I put it off for months.

Finally dragging myself to the mall, I lingered outside the lingerie store, debating if I wanted to go in. The tall, lean mannequins modeled the latest wonder bras, enticing shoppers with their sculpted bodies and perfectly shaped breasts. I felt a wave of jealousy, surprised to realize I had sunk so low as to be envious of a dummy. What had happened to my healthy body image? My confidence as a woman?

Taking a deep breath, I walked in. Soon I found myself standing half naked under the unforgiving dressing room lights, a rainbow of bras stacked on the bench beside me. The bully waltzed in. He latched the door shut as he leaned close, his breath foul.

"Freak," he whispered.

I touched the puckered edges of the scars. With the mirrors flanking me on all sides, I felt like I had stepped into a fun house at the fair. As a child, I laughed at the weird shapes and sizes of my reflection in those fun houses.

I wasn't laughing that day.

My hands trembled as I chose a vivid blue bra with matching lace trim. The fabric was soft and delicate. I adjusted the straps and hooked the back. I flexed my body, as I turned this way and that.

"Damaged," the bully chortled.

His lies were familiar. I had heard them as a pimply faced teenager and later as a new mom coming to terms with a body that wouldn't squeeze back into prepregnancy jeans. I had not expected to hear them again at my age.

"Ugly," the bully taunted.

I examined my living, breathing, cancer-fighting body. I shook my head. "Beautiful," I said. I heard the truth in my own words. Truth I hadn't realized my mother had taught me with her ever-present lipstick. Truth that had nothing to do with the bra I modeled.

Truth I had seen in the eyes of many cancer survivors. Truth I wanted others to know.

Cancer may take and take and try to strip you down as you bare your skin again and again to strangers who stare at you with clinical eyes. You may feel reduced to a number in a medical file as you lie again on an examining table, but believe me when I tell you this: you are beautiful.

You—without hair and eyelashes. You are beautiful.

You—with the chemo rash and the nausea. You are beautiful.

You—without breasts but with a body covered in scars. You are beautiful.

And maybe you are not a cancer survivor, but you know what it's like to live in a world that takes and takes and strips you of who you are. You have heard the voice of a lie that says you are nobody.

You. You are beautiful.

Grab your tube of lipstick—not as a symbol of movie-star glamour but of choosing to take control of the things you can. Reclaim your beauty. Reestablish your God-given identity. Slide off the cap. Apply the color first to your top lip. Then the bottom. Purse your lips together. Clean off that smudge in the corner with a tissue.

Now smile. Take back your lunch money.

Cancer has taken my mom's hair and eyebrows, the contents of her stomach, and has sent her to the hospital again and again, but it turns out cancer is not so powerful after all.

Cancer cannot strip away femininity.

Cancer cannot erase God-given purpose and destiny.

Cancer cannot steal beauty.

Mom proves it again and again—every time she grabs her lipstick.

Twenty-three

When Foundations Shake

The sun is slipping behind the peaks of the Estrellas overlooking the lands of the Gila River Reservation. Kevin and I pull into the dirt lot at the trailhead on one of the many paths of the South Mountain Preserve, the largest municipal park in the nation.

Temperatures are predicted to fall to thirty-one degrees, so we stuff light jackets into our day packs, along with our usual first aid kit, granola bars, and water. We laugh, because in the confusion of giving last-minute instructions about oxygen levels and pain meds to our daughter Aleah, both of us grabbed matches, but neither one of us thought to bring a headlamp. Sunset is in twenty-four minutes, and we plan on a four-mile hike.

We click the leash on Mollie and head for the Bursera Trail at a fast pace. We pass creosote and cactus, no blossoms splashing color on the dusty landscape as we go chasing daylight.

As we head west on the ridgeline, the first blush of color paints the sky over the peak in front of us. My husband points to a crumbled ruin nestled into the mountain, off to our right.

"It's interesting what appears in different light," Kevin says.

The ruin, tucked into the hillside, is known as the Lost Ranch. It's often camouflaged in bright sunlight, but the waning sun highlights one of two old stone fireplaces, the hearth a dark cavern in the final rays. The ranch predates the establishment of the park in 1924, but the true reason for a building without road access remains a mystery. Ahwatukee Foothills historian Marty Gibson pondered this in an article: "What was the approximately two-thousand-square-foot structure in its heyday—and when may that have been? Could the building have been a private residence? A miners' camp? Perhaps a government work project? No one, including the rangers, seems to know. Public records which might explain the circumstances, background or intent of the structure and whoever built it are seemingly non-existent. What is certain is that long ago, someone went to a lot of trouble to build a structure that has partially survived well beyond its original intended purpose. An air of mystery prevails."[1]

I glance over my shoulder as we continue to ascend the ridgeline. Besides the fireplaces, a section of flooring and most of the foundation remain. Five crumbling steps open to the mountains that flank the ruins on three sides. The golden light bounces off the nearly century-old foundation as the ending of another day warms the rough stonework.

I agree with my husband. It is curious what can be seen in different light and to discover what is visible in the final beams of daylight.

I can't help but remember another set of ruins: the ruins of Machu Picchu in Peru that we visited after Dad died. From the moment we entered the ruins in the early morning while a slight drizzle fell, we were captivated. Only the waking birds broke the silence as we first viewed the Inca civilization shrouded in mist swirling up from the Urubamba River valley. We felt like we had stepped into a scene from *The Lord of the Rings*, with us as the actors, transported back to another moment in time.

I wondered what American explorer Hiram Bingham felt when he came to the site in 1911. Bingham had gone seeking the lost city of Vilcabamba, the last stronghold of the Incas, when he was led to Machu Picchu by a few locals, including a man who promised to show Bingham the ruins if he was paid fifty cents for his day's wage.[2]

Although now excavated, Machu Picchu still remains largely a mystery. Was it a royal retreat or country palace? Was it a normal Inca city—a political, religious, and administrative center? Was it a trade center with its eight access routes radiating out into the jungle? Without any historical documents to answer these questions, archaeologists have to read what the Incas left behind—the stones, artifacts, and mummies—to find the answers.

Built in the fifteenth century, the genius of the engineering that went into building Machu Picchu still enthralls engineers today. "My reaction was one of admiration, one of awe, because these people did not have a written language, they did not have iron or steel, they did not use the wheel, and yet they were . . . good. And we know they were good because Machu Picchu has lasted for some 500 years,"[3] said Kenneth R. Wright, a hydrologist and civil engineer who has studied the water works and engineering achievements of Machu Picchu since 1994.

According to our Quechuan guide, Hiram Bingham labeled one wall in Machu Picchu "the most beautiful wall in the Americas" because of its exceptional design and the way the stones were shaped and carved. Centuries later, the wall still stands, having withstood the wear and tear of seventy-six inches of rain every year for over five centuries. Many of the stones are still so tight a credit card cannot be slid between the cracks.

The walls of Machu Picchu, built over two fault lines, are also no stranger to earthquakes. Seismically, Peru is an unstable country. Both Lima and Cusco have been damaged by earthquakes in the past. How could the walls of Machu Picchu still be standing?

One answer is dancing stones.

The stones are cut and wedged together without the use of mortar. According to a National Geographic website, "When an earthquake occurs, the stones in the Inca buildings are said to dance, that is, they bounce through the tremors and then fall back into place. Without this building method, many of the best known buildings at Machu Picchu would have collapsed long ago."[4]

Dancing stones are not the only mystery at Machu Picchu.

As many as twenty-five hundred people a day come to view the mysterious stone ruins of Machu Picchu that exist above the ground. But 50–60 percent of the Incan engineers' work was done below the surface. An excavation near the plaza found that the prepared foundation goes down nine feet, including three feet of topsoil, then a layer of sandy/gravelly soil, and finally, a drainage layer made up of leftover waste rock.[5]

The same can be said about the agricultural terraces that are held in place by stone retaining walls. The terraces have the same subsurface drainage, with a layer of stones at the bottom, followed by gravel, sandy material, and topsoil.[6] The centuries-old foundation keeps the mystery of Machu Picchu from eroding down the mountainside when it is bombarded by the elements.

When the mountains shake, Machu Picchu remains because of its foundation.

———

Back on the ridgeline in Arizona, my husband and I snap photos of the sunset and jog back to the car. Mars is visible over the Estrellas when we make it back to the trailhead. Behind us the red lights of the radio towers on South Mountain blink their warning. I can no longer see the old ruin of the Lost Ranch, but I know it is there, the foundation stones holding together in the darkness.

Nighttime is upon us.

———

Mom is back in the hospital. After numerous tests, a CT scan reveals another blood clot in her right lung—this while on baby aspirin and two blood thinners. A condition, tied to her cancer, causes her blood to clot. Her breathing is compromised.

"The cancer has moved to her lungs," the pulmonologist surmises.

"Your mom has pneumonia," the oncologist suggests.

It's a game of "red rover" and neither wants to call Mom over to his team.

While the two experts debate treatment options, I only know one thing: Mom wants yogurt. Strawberry. By the time she is settled, it is long past dinnertime.

I take the elevator to the hospital cafeteria, located in the basement of the facility. The foundation of the hospital is food, a notion that makes complete sense to me.

In our growing-up years, Mom was never one for fancy meals; she was more a meat, potatoes, veggies, and a slab of butter on white bread type of cook—with a bowl of canned peaches for dessert. The first food Mom taught me to make was baking powder biscuits, light and fluffy, served with melted butter and homemade strawberry jam. And now, we are full circle, Mom sitting at my table, requesting baking powder biscuits after chemo.

As I step into the hospital basement, my senses are bombarded by the aromas of chicken soup, pepperoni pizza, and a hundred days of reheated chili. The door to the cafeteria is locked.

I am not concerned, because I know the hospital has a vending machine stocked with fruit and other nutritious snacks. As I peer through the glass door, I am thrilled to see there is strawberry yogurt. A handwritten sign is taped to the machine: "Cash only."

I put away my credit card and dig through my purse. I only have a twenty. I need $1.50 for the yogurt.

Thankfully, there is a change machine next to the vending machine. I stuff in my twenty. The machine spits it back out. The machine is broken.

The dominoes keep toppling, and it is too much.

Too much.

The last bit of light sinks behind the clouds. I stand on a crumbling foundation as my world shakes. I know I should remind myself of God's past goodness and faithfulness. I know I should pray or believe—or something.

193

"With the kind You show Yourself kind," the psalmist writes in Psalm 18:25. Other versions say faithful. Or merciful.

I stare at my haggard face reflected in the vending machine door. Hasn't Mom deposited enough coins of kindness to deserve at least a yogurt out of the deal? What more is required?

I remember Mom telling stories of going every Sunday until she was sixteen to a little country church where Norwegian was spoken. Of taking a horse and sleigh across the fields to get there in the winter. Of a Christmas Eve service around a candlelit tree, including two ushers who stood by with pails of water "just in case." Of coming home from that service with a paper lunch bag filled with peanuts, hard candies, and an orange. She was at the church with her family whenever the doors were open.

"I accepted Jesus as my Savior when I was in eighth grade," Mom once told me. "I was in a Lutheran boarding school away from home. I made the decision during the first spiritual emphasis week at a chapel service."

I do the math in my head. Eighth grade. Age thirteen. Sixty-five years ago.

With the kind You show Yourself kind? With the faithful You show Yourself faithful? Merciful?

I slap the vending machine with the palm of my hand. Tears blur my vision as I zip my purse closed and turn toward the elevator.

A man taps me on the shoulder. I wonder how long he has been watching me crumble, my face distraught and my mascara raining down.

Before I can find words to explain myself, he drops something into my hand and walks away.

I open the fingers of my slapping, angry hand, still red and trembling.

In my palm are six quarters.

What do you do when cancer continues to come with seismic shaking? When it continues to come and try to take it all?

Mom fights hard not to let cancer define her beauty as she wears her earrings and places her lipstick on the tray next to her hospital bed. As cancer continues to strip her down, she reveals what is her foundation. Or more important, who.

I remember a receptionist at the doctor's office in Mom's hometown in Minnesota who came around her desk to talk to me and my sister when Mom had left the waiting room.

"I have had my own issues of loss," the receptionist said, "but I have watched your mother all these months and have watched her deal with her loss with such grace." Her voice faded as she cleared her throat.

"I need to relook at my own anger issues with God," the woman said.

My mother, who welcomes doctors into their own exam rooms, has this effect on people.

Romans 2:4 says it is the kindness of God that leads people to repentance. Did you catch that?

Kindness can lead people to gaze once again into the face of God.

Mom holds not only a tube of lipstick in her hand, but she also holds a key. She, who is Christ's hands and feet on this earth, has the ability to open the door to lead people back to God. That key is kindness.

Proverbs 3:3 states, "Do not let kindness and truth leave you; bind them around your neck, write them on the tablet of your heart."

When we find ourselves hit from all sides. When we find our foundation smashed again and again. When we find ourselves living in our own fault zone. We must. We must hold tightly to that key. We can't place it on the dresser or tuck it away in a back drawer. We must hang it around our necks, because kindness can be so easily lost.

In its place we are left with bitterness. Disappointment. Cynicism. Crumbling stones.

Beth Moore writes, "Often when someone we know is in need, our feelings of inadequacy paralyze us. We know we can't fix the problem, so we remain distant. Our lack of power may keep us from exercising the lesser power we possess."[7]

Back in Mom's hospital room, I struggle with these feelings of paralyzing inadequacy. Feeling utterly powerless, what lesser power could I possibly possess?

Timely kindness.[8]

"Do not withhold good . . . when it is in your power to act" (Prov. 3:27 NIV). Sometimes the desire to do a great thing (fix the entire problem), keeps us from doing a good thing (be kind in a small way).

The stranger at the vending machine couldn't erase the blood clot in Mom's right lung. He couldn't cure her from metastatic ovarian cancer. He couldn't even fix the broken change machine or buy me a four-course dinner. But he could give me six quarters.

While my foundation shook, he exercised his lesser power of timely kindness.

He could have stepped back because he couldn't do the great thing. Instead, he stepped forward and did the good thing. He could have judged my darkness, but instead, he chose to step into the remaining rays of light and became the kindness of Christ to me as I felt the stones shake beneath my soul's foundation on an earthquaking day.

In our culture, we have forgotten the meaning of kindness. We picture it on the list of polite manners, right up there with using a knife to cut your food and covering your mouth when you sneeze. But we have lost the sense of kindness having transformational power, of kindness turning people to repent.

I know.

Six quarters caused me to turn my face, once again, to my Jesus who loves.

Who loves.

Who loves.

Twenty-four

The Gethsemane Hour

Water.

One singular thought throbbed in my brain and rolled off my tongue, thick and dry in the scorching Arizona heat.

I needed water.

After almost three decades of hiking in the desert, I struggled to believe on that day several years ago that we were nearly out of fluids. Jokes about it being a dry heat ended several miles ago. Complaints about the hiking website being wrong dwindled to silence.

We trudged along under the relentless sun—my husband, son, daughter-in-law, daughter, and I—our feet kicking up desert dust on a trail edged with creosote bushes and prickly pear—survivors in the desert that takes no prisoners.

I glanced over my shoulder. My daughter-in-law's lips flattened in a grim line, a white line of dried sweat above her lips. My son's shoulders hunched as he conserved energy inward. My daughter limped from a sprained ankle. Weariness replaced determination.

Behind them, the Catalina Mountains near Tucson, Arizona, stood sentinel, the promising shade too far away for relief. The mountains had been touted on the website as the perfect backdrop for viewing desert flowers, wildlife, and cactus. Posted photos of desert daisies and blooming paloverde had enticed us to leave our air-conditioned vehicle at the trailhead. We had thrown on day packs for what was supposed to be a short adventure.

The website was incorrect.

We were in trouble.

We were not novices. Our hiking boots had logged countless miles on desert trails. We knew the simple rule—you always pack more water than you think you need. We had not counted on wrong information and a sprained ankle.

The point was moot as we plodded step after weary step.

In the distance we saw a group of teens sitting near a young mesquite tree, the narrow trunk offering a slice of shade. Boy Scouts! Surely they came prepared with water to share! Our pace quickened with our hope of water.

All too soon we discovered they had read the same website and were also low on fluids. Our heat-fried brains delivered morbid tales of vultures and skeletons as we soberly confronted our joint idiocy. Besides not packing adequate water, we made one other grave mistake—we allowed our past knowledge and experience to lull us into complacency. Years of living in desert suburbia had erroneously made us believe we understood all about desert living. Instead, we found ourselves under the blazing sun with no relief in sight.

We discussed options.

"Some of us should go ahead," my husband said. "We have supplies in the car and can bring them back."

I fantasized about the gallon jug of warm water in the car. If there had been a drop of moisture left in my mouth, I would have salivated. I craved every ice cube I had ever carelessly dumped down the sink. A Scout leader joined my husband and son and they jogged down the trail.

I sucked on the hose of my water pack. After one tiny sip of water, I was left with only air. My container was bone dry. I remembered the water I had used at the beginning of the hike to wet my warm face and neck. How I longed for that water!

I was so thirsty.

The sky was cloudless. Shadeless. With blasting sun at its pinnacle, our shadows melted off us into little gray puddles at our feet. The spines of the surrounding prickly pear and ocotillo offered no respite or welcome.

We could not escape.

Pain unrelenting. Merciless. Beating down with piercing brightness. Or rather, darkness. A floor doc changes Mom's pain meds without talking to me. Mom spirals to a dark, excruciating place.

Morphine does *nothing*!

I walk into Mom's hospital room—into the full-blown heat of pain with no escape. In the stark, stripped-bare reality, no comfort can be found. No narrow width of shadow.

I never knew a clock could tick so slowly.

"Relax and breathe," the nurse says to Mom. She speaks quietly while she massages Mom's fingers. I remember, years ago, the soothing voice of a labor nurse who did the same for me at the birth of our second daughter, while I struggled to bring her into the world.

Perhaps we all need healing touch at the changing of worlds.

"Close your eyes," the nurse instructs. "Concentrate on my voice. That's it. Breathe in slowly while I count to ten."

I watch the second hand on the wall clock tick off the numbers.

"Now exhale slowly. Concentrate on my voice."

The second hand makes its circular round.

"Good. Relax and breathe. The doctor will be here soon."

The nurse continues counting and breathing for several minutes. Some of the pinched look leaves Mom's face.

"Can I come in?" a friend asks from the doorway.

"Yes," I say, low and desperate, grabbing his life preserver arm.

"This looks like a bad time," he says. He steps back, unsure, while I tug him into a shadeless room.

"It's a horrible, no-good morning," I admit, no longer caring that tears are running down my face.

I notice tears in his eyes and remember he is still new in his grief from the death of his wife from this wretched disease. He grips my shoulder and stands beside me as we watch my mother breathe, both of us with no more words.

I remember twenty-five years ago when Mom came to visit after we lost a baby in the second trimester of pregnancy. We sat at my kitchen table and talked about the loss of our much-wanted daughter and her granddaughter. Mom began to cry.

"I'm so sorry," she said.

"Sorry?" I questioned. "For what? Loving me enough to feel my pain?"

"Weep with those who weep" (Rom. 12:15), Paul encourages. One of the names of Jesus in Isaiah 53:3 is "man of sorrows." In the face of another's pain, I often allow myself to become paralyzed in my fear of doing or saying the wrong thing. At times I have wanted to tidy the chaos of another's story, to interrupt as they stutter over the sentences that are all about upheaval.

With the arm of my older friend around me, I realize it's not about finding the perfect words. It's not about "do" or "say." It's about dropping the perfect and simply being in the mess.

Sometimes tears are the bravest gift we give.

We are in the Gethsemane Hour, pleading, "May this cup pass from me."[1]

This cup of suffering and loss, a finish line of faith we would not have chosen. And I ask, like Jesus asked, *Will you tarry, linger, wait? Take your time leaving?*

Will you remain with me and not give me medical advice or an article on the advantages of cooking with kale?

Will you wait and not stick a religious platitude on my gaping wound? Will you not be in a hurry to leave?

Will you sit without answers, yet be brave enough to listen silently to my burning questions?

Will you hang out with me for one hour, in the broken, in the dying, in the pain, in the suffering?

Will you join me in knee-bent agony, as I whisper, "Not my will, but Yours be done"?

Will you be beside me when angels come and minister?

"Can you read Psalm 91?" Mom asks, her voice thin. Strained.

"'He who dwells in the secret place of the Most High,'" I recite from memory.

"'Shall abide under the shadow of the Almighty,'" Mom whispers.

Mom and I hold hands and pray to the Almighty. We pray He will hide Mom in His secret place of shadow, within the shade of His protecting presence.

"Amen," Mom whispers when the pleading words run out.

I do not sense His presence among the beeping monitors, on the sweat-beaded forehead of my mother.

But He is not absent.

I find Him in my older friend who, after standing with me at Mom's bedside for a few minutes, goes to sit in the hall. He decides to stay until the crisis has passed, praying for two hours while medical staff steps around him. He rips out a page from his Bible because he has no other paper with which to leave me a handwritten, encouraging prayer.

I find Him in a friend who brings lunch and another who arranges meals for our family. I find Him in a friend who delivers homemade Norwegian cookies. In another who comes and sits with me.

I see Him in countless people who pray and send messages from Norway, Minnesota, Arizona, California, Colorado, South America, and across an online community.

I see Him, so clearly, in the nurse who arrived in the middle of the mess at the shift change and says, "I will fix it" and works until the pain is gone. I discover Him in an unknown doctor who walks into the room, whom I cry all over, who says, "I will take full responsibility," and prescribes Mom the meds she needs.

I discover Him in my husband, who drops everything and comes to be with me at the hospital. And in my kids, who rearrange Mom's bedroom to make room for a hospital bed. In my siblings, who call and fly into town, making me feel grateful I am not an only child.

I find Him in community.

"I was sick and you visited me," the Bible records in Matthew 25:36 (ESV). I always considered the statement something nice to do, like sending a thank-you note for a present or returning the shopping cart to the cart corral at the grocery store. The practice is much more than *nice*. I realize that on an entirely different level.

When we visit, stand without words, share tears, write a card, send an inquiring text or phone call, utter prayers, bring a meal, drive someone to an appointment, or extend a hand in mercy, we are not simply being nice.

No, we are doing so much more.

On a horrible, spiraling-into-the-pit, painful day, my lifelines are friends and family who constantly checked on us and the medical staff who works tirelessly to care for Mom. Just as my husband and son were able to bring back water to us that day we ran out of it in the desert, this community comes bearing a cup of cold water to my liquid-deprived soul.

In that compassion, I do not find nice. I discover the answer to our prayer.

"He that dwelleth in the secret place of the most High shall abide under the shadow of the Almighty."[2]

I found the shade of God.

Twenty-five

An Ordinary Life

"I have no magic pill to offer," Mom's oncologist says.

"I know," Mom replies. Sometimes courage puts on a favorite purple scarf and sits in a cancer facility.

"We are running out of options."

"Yes."

"It's time to focus on quality of life. On unfinished business."

This conversation starts several days of thinking, praying, and questioning.

"I am done," Mom says to me.

"Done? No more items on the list?" I am aware that seeing her great-grandbabies and visiting my brother at Christmas were two items on her list. Both have been completed.

Mom shakes her head. Tired of fighting. Done.

What is it like for a master list-maker to be finished? On her computer are the following files, the following lists: *The Improvements We've Made to the Property List. The Address, Email, Birthday, and Phone Number List* of the 412 descendants from an extended family reunion she planned for her side of the family. *The Vehicles We've Owned List. The Christmas Gifts We've Given the Grandchildren*

List. And a six-page, two-columned, single-spaced *Inventory List* of practically every item still at the Minnesota acreage, including the barn, outbuildings, and a two-level home with complete basement—with an additional file of photos of each item.

My memories of Mom before her stroke are of a whirling dynamo, a woman who put the Energizer bunny to shame. Her organizing, serving, list-making, doing personality defined her. Then the stroke. Outwardly, it appears she has lost no motor skills, but writing remains difficult. Typing? Impossible. Making lists is an arduous task. She literally has to draw out the words on the page with her finger and then attempt to use a pen. Sometimes the scribbles are undecipherable.

As the cancer has progressed, even the lists Mom keeps in her brain have shortened. Become silent. Doing no longer defines her. She concentrates on being.

From her life, a beautiful, queenly graciousness has emerged. Maybe it has been there all along, but it was masked in the doing. Cancer has removed the mask. There in the midst of suffering is beauty in the being—displayed for everyone to see.

In an episode of the TV series *Doctor Who*, the doctor travels forward in time with the painter Vincent van Gogh. The doctor asks an art museum curator for his opinion of the painter's work. The curator extols van Gogh's command of color, then adds, "[Van Gogh] transformed the pain of his tormented life into ecstatic beauty. Pain is easy to portray, but to use your passion and pain to portray the ecstasy and joy and magnificence of our world, no one had ever done it before."[1]

Pain and suffering in itself has no glory. Portraying pain is easy. I don't know anyone who would choose such an existence. Most cancer patients I know who are applauded for being inspirational and brave would say, "I don't want to be a hero. I just want to grow older." Yet finding beauty in life, despite the pain, is what shouts so loudly. This choice makes it possible to point a seeking world to a God who loves.

In the book *A Path through Suffering*, author Elisabeth Elliot writes, "The world still needs to be shown that there are those who, no matter what the circumstances, will, for love of Him, do exactly what God commands."[2] As an example, Elliot points to Christ, and paraphrases John 14:30–31: "The Prince of this world approaches. He has no rights over me; but the world must be shown that I love the Father, and do exactly as he commands."[3]

Jesus always pointed to His Father, even in the midst of suffering. Through all Mom suffers, she turns the mirror and reflects Christ.

"I have seen great beauty of spirit in some who were great sufferers," C. S. Lewis writes. "I have seen (people), for the most part, grow better not worse with advancing years, and I have seen the last illness produce treasures of fortitude and meekness from most unpromising subjects."[4]

I do not view Mom as an unpromising subject, but I have seen this great beauty of spirit in the midst of suffering as she points others to the One she loves. Friends ask in the Song of Solomon, "Who is this coming up from the desert, leaning on her beloved?" (Song of Sol. 8:5 ISV). Mom might not be walking as straight as she did in the past, and maybe she needs a walker, but she is leaning closer to her Jesus as she comes up from the desert.

What is it like to no longer have items on a bucket list? On a to-do list? For a woman who has been known for extensive, detailed lists, this is an incredible question. What is it like to be done?

When faced with the end of her life, how do the accomplishments measure up for my mom in a culture that defines life in terms of the extraordinary? Would her life be considered successful by today's exciting, risk-taking standards? Many people create bucket lists, but usually these lists are filled with finding excitement "out there."

Books like *1000 Places to See before You Die*, *1001 Guitars to Dream of Playing before You Die*, and even *1001 Books to Read before You Die* encourage the mind-set that adventure is found only in escaping current reality. Never mind that nobody has time to do a thousand of anything. Even in the church we are guilty of pushing this goal, making the focus more on faith as an adventure, rather than a life of sacrifice. After all, Jesus walked on water. Shouldn't we? I am still waiting for the book *1000 Things to Do Like Jesus before You Die.*

I sit by the hospital bedside of my mother and realize purpose and fulfillment are found right now. In this moment. In these circumstances. The biggest adventure is found in living an ordinary life in a Christlike way.

For years Mom gave me a kitchen towel tucked in with other birthday gifts, a tradition I found rather odd yet complementary to Mom's organizational style that likes the sink spotless, the table crumbless, and the dishes dried and put away. Mom wielded an effective towel.

Oswald Chambers was intrigued by the use of a towel—specifically a towel in the hands of Christ. "The things that Jesus did were of the most menial and commonplace order and this is an indication that it takes all God's power in me to do the most commonplace things in His way," Oswald writes. "Can I use a towel as He did?"[5]

Chambers refers to the passage found in John 13 when Jesus knew His final hour on this earth was approaching. Running out of earthly time, He didn't preach another sermon or heal another sick person; He picked up a towel. He didn't tuck it around some birthday gifts; He tucked it around his disciples' dirty feet, forever settling the question of how one's final days should be lived out. While wrapped in the ordinary, Jesus did the extraordinary with twelve ordinary men. In one small country. With a life cut short (by worldly standards), He fulfilled all the purposes of God.

I watch my mother sleeping, her chest rising and falling, and I contemplate bucket lists and extraordinary versus ordinary lives. I jot down a final list for Mom, a woman who stayed married to one man for fifty-five years, while living in the same house for a half century in a farming community outside of Albert Lea, Minnesota.

Lived the life she wanted. *Check.*

Found God. *Check.*

Loved one man well. *Check.*

Mothered four incredible children (if I must say so myself). *Check.*

Surrounded herself with caring friends. *Check.*

Influenced five generations during her lifetime. *Check.*

Responded with grace under pressure while wearing lipstick. *Check.*

Rich beyond measure. *Double check.*

May I live such an ordinary life.

———

Decades ago I stood on a running track, swallowing nerves that were trying to consume me whole. I concentrated on my breathing. In and out. In and out. With my arms extended in front of me, I high-stepped my legs, trying to touch my knees to my outstretched palms. My cleats clicked on the asphalt. I shook the tension out of each leg. Each arm. I rolled my neck. I brought my shoulders to my ears and lowered them in a rush of air.

"Runners take your mark."

I heard the words echo across the field, from the starting line one hundred meters away. I could barely see the first runners of the 4 × 100 relay getting into position, my teammate in lane four. It had been many years since girls from our school had made it to the Minnesota State Track and Field Championship. I felt the weight of that time.

"Set."

I loosened my arms. My legs. Again.

The sound of the starter's pistol reverberated in my ears. Clear. Sharp. In a little more than twelve seconds, my teammate would come around the bend.

I located a piece of athletic tape on the track, marking my starting position right outside the exchange zone—the stretch of track where the baton must be passed from the incoming to the outgoing runner.

I knew the 4 × 100 was not simply about teaming the four fastest runners together; the race was won or lost in the passing of the baton.

I flexed my fingers. Let out my breath.

Peering over my shoulder, I saw my teammate hit her piece of tape, the predetermined spot we had found after hours and hours of practice. I took off running in the acceleration zone, ten meters outside the exchange, knowing I had about seven steps to reach my maximum speed before receiving the baton. The area is nicknamed the "fly zone" for a reason.

"Stick."

My left arm shot back, palm up, hand fully extended, close to shoulder height. I was running full out, but my arm didn't waver. My responsibility was to have a still hand, not to go grasping for what I couldn't see. Her responsibility was to place the baton. If we dropped it, we would lose the race.

I felt the smooth metal in my palm and closed my fingers tight. The baton was mine. My cleats hit the asphalt in practiced rhythm. In the distance, I could see my next teammate. Waiting.

I ran like my life depended on it.

———

The race is won or lost in the exchanging of the baton. I have found this to be true. Not only in track and field, but in life. Over the years, I have stood on that track numerous times, waiting for my mom to come around the corner. I've stood outside the acceleration zone, waiting for her to hit that predetermined spot on the track so I could fly.

I stood on the track at eighteen, when Mom helped me pack my suitcase, tucking in extra wool socks next to the jeans and long underwear. "Live your dreams," Mom said as my palm closed around the smooth metal. I took off running.

A few years later, Mom stood on one side of me and Dad on the other, and they escorted me down the aisle of a church crowded with wedding guests. They placed my hand in the hand of my soon-to-be husband. Mom adjusted my veil and kissed my cheek. "God bless you," she whispered as I turned and ran the next leg of my journey.

Later, when I held my first child, Mom made the trip as soon as she could manage it on her teacher's schedule. Food appeared on the table like magic, dirty dishes disappeared from the sink, and she declared her grandson (and each subsequent grandchild) the most amazing ever.

Through the years, we have participated in this exchange countless times.

I find myself on the track again. There is a knowing inside me that this is the final exchange. Mom is coming once again around the bend. Cancer has taken its toll. Her silver hair fluffs in the breeze as her feet scrape along the track. Her arms shake as she pushes her red walker. Her right hand holds the walker handle, and yet, somehow, she still manages to grasp the baton.

We are in the fly zone.

I notice this baton appears heavier. Weightier. It is old and worn, as if it has traveled many miles. In fact, it has.

Mom received the baton from her mother, Lillian Clara Kloster Wika, a South Dakota farm wife who mothered twelve children. Lillian received the baton from her mother, Brynhild Christine Lande Kloster. The baton has been passed from one woman to another, throughout the generations. Brita to Christine to Brynhild to Lillian to Lois.

And now to me.

Mom readjusts her grip. This is the passing of an entire generation. When we hit the exchange zone, I will become the matriarch of the family. We are not there yet, but I sense the coming. I feel the weight of it.

On that day, my left hand will shoot back, palm up, hand fully extended, close to shoulder height. My job will be to hold still, not grasp for what I can't see. Mom's job will be to place the baton in my outstretched fingers. In that moment, her race will be done.

Mom has been preparing me for this moment my entire life—to run my race with God's strength, choosing family and faith as my feet hit the ground in practiced rhythm. My eyes focus down the track.

I see my sons in the distance. My daughters. My grandchildren.

I tighten my grip.

I run like their lives depend on it.

26

Chocolate Rain

My husband comes into Mom's bedroom as she lounges in her recliner, her feet propped up and her oxygen machine a continuous sound of life. He asks if she needs anything.

I am transported back in time to the last day of my own cancer treatment. After my final radiation, I rang the bell at the cancer clinic, took congratulatory photos with two thumbs up, ate ice cream with the family, and then decided to lie down in our bedroom. I was spent.

My husband followed me. "Is there anything you need?" he asked.

"A nap." I spread out flat on the bed.

He lingered. Even in my exhausted state, I could tell something was on his mind.

"I downloaded a song for you," he said. Unsure. Hesitant.

I propped myself on one elbow to see his face. "A song for me?"

He smiled, sheepish. "Yeah." He pulled up the song. Words of hope, a new day, and the world being okay again filled the room.

The simplicity of the words shot into a deep place in my heart I didn't even know was there. *I'm going to be okay.* For the first time I allowed myself to believe it was true. I was going to live cancer-free. I was going to beat cancer.

As I continued listening to the music, lying on the bed, with tears escaping down my cheeks, my husband picked up a bag of chocolates from his desk in the bedroom. In an unplanned bit of whimsy, he poured the candy over me. Chocolate landed in my hair. In my lap. Bounced all over the bed.

In that moment, my heart turned over for this man who had loved me through cancer, who said my scars didn't matter, who called me beautiful, who played songs of healing over me and then rained chocolates down on my head, spilling happiness everywhere.

And now . . .

This man is in a different bedroom, kneeling at the feet of a different woman, asking the same question: "Is there anything you need?"

When Kevin and I stood years ago, promising forever love, nobody told us . . . not . . . one . . . single . . . person . . . that when we spoke vows of "in sickness and in health," one day the love would encompass the "in sickness and in health" of my mother. We had no clue.

Nobody told me—or maybe I wasn't listening—that weddings and marriage and coupleness extend beyond the two to the family. Nobody told me three decades ago . . . not . . . one . . . single . . . person . . . that one day I would watch him come into Mom's room after we returned home from five days in the hospital and I would fall in love with him all over again.

Kevin kneels low to view Mom's eyes. He squeezes her hand, which is terribly bruised from a losing war with the IV needle.

"Welcome home." He smiles. Softly.

Mom smiles in return. "Thank you."

We have lived this journey through my cancer and the cancer of all our parents, during which time I have been stupid strong and we both have been clueless as we sojourned an unknown trail through the desert, a trail of more questions than answers, of mystery and suffering. And now we face—together—the reality that Mom is done.

A different done.

Occasionally in the relationships of loving one another, we stumble into a moment so precious and priceless it takes your breath away, for you catch a glimpse of what God's love is really like. In that moment you find yourself mingling with the Divine.

When you come face-to-face with God's love, your heart turns over. He walks with you through your darkest hour. He says your scars don't matter, because you are beautiful. He sings songs of healing over you and then rains blessings down on your head, spilling out happiness everywhere.

And when you are done and have fought the good fight, He kneels and looks you in the eyes and says, "Welcome home."

Twenty-seven
The Better Offer

When I was a young girl, Mom and Dad led backpacking trips to the Bighorn Mountains of Wyoming with youth from our church. We kids would stay with friends or relatives for ten days while our parents headed to the mountains. Lightweight tents had recently appeared on the market, replacing heavy canvas models, but were too expensive. So Mom and a group of ladies sewed dozens of two-man tents from mustard yellow ripstop nylon.

Years after the trips ended, Mom still held on to several tents. The memories of all those sewing hours rendered the camping gear too valuable to throw away. Even after the basement flooded and the tents mildewed and the waterproofing wore off, Mom refused to throw them out. Instead, she tried to convince each of us—her children—to take them. When that didn't work, she started on the grandchildren.

No amount of persuasion could get Mom to throw away her tents. In her opinion, holding tightly to them was the only option. We could not come up with a better offer.

I walk into the hospice facility where Mom has been transferred. Three days have passed since she declared she was done. I arrive to agony.

I have seen Mom in pain many times before, the worst being, ironically, the times I have taken her to the hospital, when they have messed with her meds. We estimated her pain level then to be an eight, maybe a nine.

I never wanted to see a ten.

I am seeing a ten now.

A relentless, searing, color-devouring ten. Another blood clot. A pulmonary embolism. All else fades under the piercing burn.

I want to be a little girl and sit on the end of the bed and have Mom comfort me, in this, a living nightmare. *Mommy, I'm scared. Can you sing a song with me? A song in the night?*

Instead, I do what she asked me to do. I become her voice when she can no longer be a voice. I talk with the nurse about pain meds. I hold Mom's hand. Do the comforting. I call siblings. Leave messages.

I call my husband. "Please come. Right away."

My husband arrives with our daughter Katelyn. Kevin takes one glance at Mom, kneels, and begs God for mercy.

I collapse on the corner of Mom's bed. Squeeze her hands, her fingers covered in rings. I rotate her wedding ring. The night before, our daughter Aleah talked to Mom about her rings as she sat with her through the night. Five rings—her wedding ring, a ring with the gemstones of her four kids, a ring with her December birthstone, a ring of hearts from Bogota, Colombia—the location of a mission my parents supported for years—and a ring of Black Hills gold from her birthplace in South Dakota.

I can't imagine Mom's hands without her rings. "Hands," according to Aleah, "that have seen so much life and love. Hands that have worked so hard and prayed so long." Hands with fingers now trembling.

Mom cannot focus on the nurse. On my husband. On her granddaughter. On me. She focuses on One. The One who loves her most.

The pain and cancer, to the very end, are trying to define her, to put parameters on her loving. On her believing. On her existence. Cancer, once again, seeks to steal all the words.

She, still the most brave, will have none of that. Through gritted teeth, she speaks what defines her. *Who* defines her.

"Jesus. Jesus." She repeats His name again and again.

A plea. A prayer. A clinging. A call to her dear friend.

The pain attempts to drown her, but she sees Him, the One who loves her most, coming to her in the storm. He is not a ghost. He has come to escort her through the narrow place.

I feel—sense—a pressing on my shoulder. I hear words.

"This is a momentary, light affliction."

The words do not come from my husband. From any other person in the room. The words come from within. From the One who loves *me* most.

"This is a momentary, light affliction."

I hear the words. I can't believe I am hearing the words. If a person had spoken these words to me—right here, right now—I would have punched them in the nose.

Momentary? Light? I experience neither of those realities, yet I hear the truth in words that wash deep. Written words, memorized, speak to me of the living Word, Jesus, who is with us in the room. Death is not the biggest shadow. Jesus, in all the difficult beauty, is larger.

> For momentary, light affliction is producing for us an eternal weight of glory far beyond all comparison, while we look not at the things which are seen, but at the things which are not seen; for the things which are seen are temporal, but the things which are not seen are eternal.
>
> For we know that if the earthly tent which is our house is torn down, we have a building from God, a house not made with hands, eternal in the heavens. . . . For indeed while we are in this tent, we groan, being burdened, because we do not want to be unclothed but to be clothed, so that what is mortal will be swallowed up by life. (2 Cor. 4:17–5:4)

Love
slipped into the room
in the place of the dying.
With fierce determination,
Love
gripped the hand of suffering,
whispering,
"I have not forgotten you.
You will not die alone."
Today
in the place of the dying,
Love kept that promise.

Mom, the woman who once sewed tents, is ready to exchange hers for a permanent dwelling. Her tent—so damaged. The water-proofing gone. The zipper torn. Cancer between the seams.

Mom finally has the better offer. We watch as all that is mortal is swallowed up before our eyes with life. Beautiful, everlasting life.

Twenty-eight
No More Good-Byes

Coo-OO-coo-oo. Coo-OO-coo-oo. The mourning dove laments on the trail, the dawn not yet birthed to light. Mollie's ears perk up, hoping the bird will provide a more interesting adventure than the neighborhood cats that torment her through the locked screen door at home. I have hit the trail early, awake again at 4:00 a.m. I cannot shake the schedule of past awakenings to give Mom her pills in the middle of the night.

The trail is gray. The surrounding rocks . . . drab. The plants appear as shadows, not real at all, only dark outlines of themselves. I stop to take a photo, lie prone on the ground that is thirsty from lack of rain. The desert dust covers my jeans and cancer survivor T-shirt. I remember the day hiking the Havasu Canyon when our daughter collapsed on the trail and refused to budge . . . one . . . more . . . inch.

"Just leave me here."

Lying here in the dryness, I echo the words. If God spoke all life into existence but then took man and breathed *life* into Adam's dust and declared His creation *very good*, and He still takes dust and makes it beautiful, I must admit I am struggling to find beauty in the remembering of my mother, the desolation in the grief of her dying.

During the months of Mom's cancer, I had pictured her last moments in my mind. The scenarios varied slightly, but I always envisioned Mom surrounded by her entire family. I didn't anticipate my siblings ready to board airplanes and not making it in time. I pictured a gentle passing. Like Dad. I thought Mom would die like Dad died. During the weeks of spiraling chaos and uncontrollable changes, I clung to the thought of this sameness.

The hardest part of grieving is rewriting the stories we have told ourselves.

The thoughts haunt my steps. I want to remain flat on my belly. *Ashes to ashes, dust to dust.* Just. Leave. Me. Here.

The dove continues his mourning as an airplane flies overhead. If my grandson were here, he would point and exclaim, "Air pane. Air pane," and today of all days, his emphasis on the second syllable would be correct.

Gray shifts to sleepy lavender, still droopy-eyed and unsure of another day. Colors emerge as I wait, shapes focus, curves and angles appear as the light plays on them. Smoky mauve. Pale blue. Soft yellow.

I shiver in the morning air and wish I had grabbed a light jacket. In the weeks since Mom's death, I have experienced grief when it is a hot, visible mess, boiling over like pasta on the stove with no lid capable of keeping it down. Today grief is cold, piercing, and deep. I wonder if I will shatter into a million shards in the icy grip of it all.

I twist Mom's wedding ring on my right hand. Sorrow stabs. Hard. Sharp. I stand, shake off the dust. I pass flowering brittlebush, the blossoms shooting through a neighboring cactus, knowing the coming spring will bring butterflies to the yellow centers. With the delay in winter rains, the wildflowers are few. Sparse.

The rise in elevation is minor, but I struggle to lift my feet as I trudge up the trail. Breathing is difficult. Grief accompanies me.

As I go over the next rise, I stop. Blink. Blink again. I cannot believe what I see.

Purple flowers. Everywhere. The flowers border desert stones. Surround the cactus. From the depths of thirsty ground, I have never seen so much purple.

The scent from a bush of desert lavender wafts upward. Perfumes my memory. Every night, before Mom would turn off the light, she would put several drops of lavender oil on her pillow. Her favorite scent enveloped her dreams.

I remain frozen in my tracks, mesmerized by what I see. People hike around me, puzzled at my stillness. Mollie whimpers and settles into the dust. I am overcome. Wave upon wave of love washes over me. With Dad, God came with baby birds. With Mom, He comes with purple flowers.

Before Mom's heart attack and stroke, while she was adjusting as a new widow with her own health struggles, she wrote to the family, "Only He knows what the future holds; I look forward to many more milestones on this earth, but He has prepared a purple room filled with flowers for me in heaven! I am thankful for each day." Dozens of bouquets arrived for her funeral last month, her memory honored in the blooming.

My legs cannot hold me and I collapse into the dust, not in despair this time, but in overwhelming love from my Jesus who continues to pursue me. With quarters. With sparrows. With people wearing skin. At a hospice bedside. With flowers. I am undone, surrounded by the enormity of love. Relentless. Personal. Passionate.

He took the time to plant an entire hillside with lavender, waiting for the day when I would hike this mountain. He left nothing to chance, orchestrating this surprise party in desert dust. He didn't just hope to reach my grieving heart. He knew the exact gift I needed in order to hear His expression of love for me. No other gardener could complete such a task as the sower and lover of my soul.

On the morning of Jesus's resurrection, before people who loved Him had heard of the miracle, Mary sat in agony by the tomb, convinced someone had stolen His body. When she saw Jesus walking in the early morning light, she thought He was a gardener.

The first person, according to John, that Jesus chose to meet was Mary. Jesus didn't chat with the angels. He didn't provide any words of comfort to the terrified guards. He didn't give any speeches that began with "fear not." He didn't round up the priests to give them an object lesson of His Father's power.[1]

He appeared to Mary. And if the first person Jesus appeared to was significant, so were the first words Jesus spoke.

Jesus had died an agonizing death after being tortured, beaten by soldiers, and nailed to a cross. Now, three days later, He had experienced life and breath returning to His cold, entombed body, the light still clinging to His warming skin. What were His first words?

Jesus asked a question: "Why are you crying?" (John 20:15 NIV). His first words after His resurrection were about tears. His first priority was addressing a woman's grief.

"Why are you crying?" The question reverberates on a desert hillside and echoes in my own heart. Jesus, known as a man of sorrows and familiar with grief, who was with me when Mom died, is with me in the dust. I do not sense the pressing of His hand or hear His words, but His love and care reverberate in an explosion of violet.

Jesus asked Mary another question: "Who is it you are looking for?" (John 20:15 NIV).

Not what. *Who.* We are all looking for who. Mary. Me. You.

I have traveled a desert of questions, seeking answers, forgetting that God doesn't always answer questions; instead, He becomes the answer. To the Israelite wanderers He became the God of endless cloud and covering shadow. *He* was the answer to their question, "Why did you bring us out to the desert to die?" *He* provided protection and guidance.

In the same way, Jesus is the answer to my question. He is who I am seeking. In the midst of the hardest reality and the uncontrollable chaos, He is the promise of steadfastness. Sameness. *Yesterday, today, and forever* sameness.

I once stood under the searching eyes of my husband before a closet full of clothes, not knowing I could only find out who I was through the revealing of who God is. And today He shows me more of Himself on a hillside clothed in purple. I picture Him organizing this day, causing seeds to hold their vow and young plants to wait to bloom until the precise moment on the calendar when I will come over the rise and find a desert decorated in lavender. This is a God who counts days, yet knows my name. This is the heart of Someone who loves. This is a God who creates mountains to show He can and plants purple flowers to show He cares. A God who can and a God who cares. This is who meets me in desert dust.

Mary did not recognize Christ until He called her by name, so I too do not recognize Him until I realize He loves and pursues in a personal way. Star Namer. World Spinner. Caretaker of Sparrows. Purple Flower Planter. Knower of Me. Knower of You.

Now, on a desert hillside, I hear Him call my name. Surrounded by the rising scent of purple lavender, I know, without any doubt or shadow, God is still making beautiful things out of dust.

"For the LORD will have compassion on Zion," Isaiah records, "have compassion on all her ruins. He will make her wilderness like Eden, and her deserts like the garden of the LORD. Joy and gladness will be found in her, thanksgiving, and the sound of singing. Sorrow and sighing will flee away" (Isa. 51:3 ISV).

He has compassion on the broken. On those who live in ruins, ruins of illness and cancer. On those who have a diagnosis spoken over their lives. He sees tears. He comforts the grieving.

I stoop to pick up a seedpod I didn't recognize. I rub the dried exterior between my fingers until it falls open, revealing tiny wild-flower seeds, each seed full of the knowledge that spring will come again to the desert. I also carry the promise—a vow by God of a future blooming.

After the funeral, we spent a day with our grandchildren in Tucson—a day filled with trains, toddler chatter, and holding a baby. A day without thoughts of oxygen tanks, doctor appointments, and setting the alarm for the next round of pain meds. Yet it was bittersweet, as I knew Mom would have loved to have been there.

She liked nothing more than to plan a family gathering. Big or small, arranging a family event put her smack-dab in the middle of her organizational giftedness.

Lists were made with sticky notes added to the revised copies. Meals were planned. Dad was sent on various errands around the property, getting ready for the onslaught of four generations.

Now we are three generations, and I ache with the missing.

As I gathered my belongings to head back home from Tucson, our two-year-old grandson grabbed his shoes and socks and followed me out the front door.

"Phoenix?" he asked.

"You need to stay with Mommy and Daddy. Another time you can come with Grandma."

He was unconvinced. "Phoenix?" he repeated.

We loaded the car, grabbed last-minute hugs, and waved good-bye. Our grandson was still standing in the driveway, clutching his shoes and socks when we drove away.

Good-byes are difficult.

Good-byes on front porches. Good-byes at hospital bedsides. Good-byes at airports. Good-byes at gravesides.

I've experienced them all. And maybe you have too. You're left standing clutching your shoes or a letter or a shirt that smells like him or a tube of lipstick she owned or dreams that won't happen, and you wonder, *Why does it hurt so much to say good-bye?*

Like author Max Lucado, I've told myself, "Death is a natural part of living."[2]

Isn't it?

No. A thousand times, no. Our hearts were not created to say good-bye. We were created for beginnings. For baby kisses. For trampoline jumping. For deep conversation. For armloads of flowers. For continual spins on the tractor through the fields. But good-byes? No.[3]

God's original design did not include a phone call in the middle of the night. A last clutching of fingers. A missed chance for a final kiss. A wedding or a graduation or a holiday with an empty place setting. Words left unspoken.

And cancer. His original plan didn't include cancer.

So where does that leave me as I deal with good-byes now?

God is planning a different ending—an event that upstages any party my mom ever planned. We who have loved Christ, who carry the seeds of promise, will fulfill His vow to us, to live again.

Foreverness. Eternity.

Each day the desert light comes out to play from the chrysalis of dawn to the unfolding wings of sunset. The desert is breathtaking because of the light. "Sunsets are more spectacular than sunrises because damp soil dries up during the heat of the day and turns to dust. The dust is stirred up into the air by the activities of people, animals, and the wind."[4]

We live in a world where everyone is waiting for the dust to settle.

When the dust settles, I will call a friend for lunch. When the dust settles, I will make a relationship right. When the dust settles, I will go after a lifelong dream. When the dust settles, I will schedule that trip I have always talked about taking. When the dust settles, I will make a career change.

This season of cancer has taught me this truth: the dust never settles. The dust is here. The dust is stirred up. Life is messy and often difficult.

And yet.

And yet.

Dust. Unsettled dust is stunning in light's revealing. Stirred up dust makes beauty possible. Desert skies need dust to paint colorful pictures.

While I stand in the dusty in-between, I am reminded that a day is coming that will be more beautiful than a thousand painted skies—when I will need His shade no longer because I will stand face-to-face in His presence. He will be the only light. "And there will be no night there—no need for lamps or sun—for the Lord God will shine on them. And they will reign forever and ever" (Rev. 22:5 NLT).

"No longer will you have the sun for light by day, nor for brightness will the moon give you light; but you will have the LORD for an everlasting light, and your God for your glory. Your sun will no longer set, nor will your moon wane; for you will have the LORD for an everlasting light, and the days of your mourning will be over" (Isa. 60:19–20).

No mourning. No shadows. No cancer. No darkness. No hiding.

I will stand free and unafraid under His glorious, pure light. In the revealing, I will know, just as I am fully known.[5] Standing with me will be all those who hung on until the end, who were not defined by *what* but chose *Who* and ran to His protecting shadow.

Cousins and grandkids. Best friends. Great-great-great-great-grandparents. Neighbors and hiking buddies. My mom and my dad. A huge rowdy bunch of in-laws and a few outlaws (remember the thief on the cross) who will join together in one humongous family gathering.

No more good-byes. No more "See you later, alligators."

As Dad said, "I will live until I die, and then my real life will begin."

Let the living begin.

Mollie woofs softly beside me. She is the first to notice. The birds have alerted her.

Two quail call to one another from opposite sides of a paloverde tree. Their typical *kwa kah kah* is shortened to one syllable. *Kah* one calls on the back side of the tree. *Kah* the other answers, like a juvenile game of Marco Polo without the swimming pool.

Mollie and I startle a small brown bird from a low creosote bush. The bird without a name flies away in a whir of complaint.

The color along the trail warms to muted brown, hinting of the coming. Plants emerge from the shadows, tossing aside their gray robes for colors of pea green, avocado, and jade.

The birds break forth in an anthem as we watch the east. I glance at my watch. Almost time.

Chirps. Tweets. Trills.

The birds cannot contain the anticipation, the heralding of the arrival. With feather and wing and voice they sing the promise.

"Here comes the sun! Here comes the sun!"

The sun crests on the horizon, golden color everywhere. The nocturnal gives way to the light.

I stand in a sunbeam and know I am not alone. So many days in the desert and I am still amazed at the most obvious beauty—the ever-present sunlight. The crowning beauty of the desert is the sun, which shines more than three hundred days a year.

Mollie and I hike along the ridgeline, the sun rising to full day behind us, displaying all the colors in the rainbow's spectrum. The yellow brittlebush. The thorny green pads on the prickly pear. The purple lavender. The sage green of the pleated saguaro. The red flash on the throat of a hummingbird.

The light bathes the stretches of sand, the ridges of canyons, and the peaks of the surrounding mountain. The colors unveil under the gathering sunlight.

The beautiful sunlight.

Note to the Reader

Thank you for joining me in my wanderings in all the difficult beautiful.

I realize that reading this story may have stirred up memories of your own sojourning in hard places. If I could, I would invite you to come with me to my favorite spot on South Mountain. We would wake early, with the night sky still in evidence. With day packs slung over our shoulders, we would hike a mile down the trail to a flat rock with a view to the horizon.

Surrounded by saguaros, brittlebush, paloverde, and the scent of creosote, we would listen to the call of the Gambel's quail and the white-winged dove, our eyes toward morning.

Here, I would listen as you told me of your own desert seasons. The dryness. The aloneness. The hard places. Maybe in your wanderings, you find yourself, like I did, redefining your views of hope, beauty, and faith.

Under a desert sky, we would whisper together of our spiritual desire for something more.

I thirst for it, don't you?

Would you consider sharing your story with me as I continue to write about hope, beauty, and faith while living in the desert? You will find me on my blog at www.lynnehartke.com.

We can wait together for the dawning.

Questions for Reflection

Since I was a little girl, I have kept a journal or diary. One of my earliest memories is sitting in the haymow of the barn drawing crayon pictures of various cats and detailing their antics in the lined notebook on my lap.

Little did I know that one day those crayon scribblings would advance into captured stories of our family's cancer journey. The book you are holding in your hands began in my journal.

Cancer was the tsunami roar that tumbled my life on its head as the waves washed over me, scrambling my emotions and beliefs on faith, hope, mortality, beauty, and purpose. For you, it may not be cancer. Perhaps your tumble is divorce. Job loss. Betrayal in a friendship. The sickness or death of someone close to you.

The circumstances that cause pain and suffering will be unique to each of us, but the need for a safe place to wade through the hard questions is common to us all. A journal can be that safe place to record thoughts and emotions that are difficult to decipher and express. Journal writing provides moments to slow down in the overwhelming flash flood of it all.

In this reflection guide, I have listed questions for each chapter to prompt you in your own storytelling as you embark on your healing journey. There is no right or wrong type of gathering stories. Some paragraphs will be a mishmash of emotions. Other pages may be philosophical. Each has value and is important as you put sentences to events larger than words on a page. Cancer, heartbreak, and trauma attempt to take many things. I pray you do not allow your words to be stolen.

It is my hope you discover, as I did, that you are not alone in this hard place but, rather, hope, beauty, and faith can be found as you hold hands in community and are pursued by a loving God.

Chapter 1: Cancer Makes a House Call

1. What memories do you have of the day tragedy, sickness, or heartbreak made a house call?
2. What do you feel has been stolen from you?
3. What questions do you have for God?

Chapter 2: Stupid Strong

1. While swimming in the pool, I decide not to allow another swimmer to finish laps before me, but in essence, I determine that the cancer diagnosis spoken over my life will not win. What memory, event, or day did you make a similar choice?
2. Do you consider yourself strong? How is that strength a positive and/or a negative thing?
3. Do you find the "why" questions mask a deeper question of "Who"?

Chapter 3: When Theology Has No Handhold

1. I use images of an upside-down map and a flash flood to put words to my difficult experience. What images do you use?

2. Do you find yourself longing for life to be "back to normal"? What aspect of "normal" have you been able to maintain? What is different?

3. I find solid ground with the truth that God is not a liar. What phrase, Scripture, or truth has helped you?

Chapter 4: I Will Live until I Die

1. Where would you place an "Add 30 Seconds" button?

2. What message do you hear when you look at the stars? Do you hear the voice of a number-loving God? Do you know you are His favorite?

3. Do you consider the boundary of time a good thing created by a loving God?

Chapter 5: Allee, Allee, All Come Free

1. When have you been surprised by unexpected emotion or grief?

2. Author Arthur W. Frank states that "illness is about learning to live with lost control." In what aspect of life has the loss of control been the most difficult for you?

3. Where do you need to be found? Where have you been hiding?

Chapter 6: Love in the Bending Low

1. Are you in a season of easy water or of collecting precious drops?

2. Ordinary life continues to happen during impossibly hard places. How do you juggle it all? How do you express love in small ways?

3. How do you struggle with soul amnesia?

Chapter 7: A Hard, Forgetting Place

1. When have you hit a "meanwhile" as you traveled from point A to point B?

2. Where do you find yourself in the pages of the story of the disciples in the boat, the storm, and Jesus coming on the waves?

3. How is your prayer life? Is it suffering? Do you look out on the waves and see only the ghost of Jesus, or do you see a dear friend?

Chapter 8: Difficult Beauty

1. How are you doing as you stand before the difficult and the beautiful? Is your heart open?

2. What do you think about the phrase "God won't give you more than you can handle"?

3. Have you discovered the wooing voice of God in the desert of Hosea 2:14?

Chapter 9: A Stack of Gratitude Stones

1. Have you experienced a magnifying glass to your emotions? What happened?

2. I write about a hike with my husband when grief wears a mask and comes out in anger. Where have you struggled with grief?

3. What three things are you grateful for today? (I would like to encourage you to take up the discipline of writing at least three things each day for which you are thankful. This practice rescued my soul from bitterness.)

Chapter 10: Laughter and Faith Hold Hands

1. When have you pushed through your own difficulties to do something important to you or to those you love?

2. What words of blessing would you speak to your family and friends?

3. On your most miserable days, are you able to hear the invitation to step off the edge of all that is known and believe in a God who loves, a God who loves, a God who loves?

Chapter 11: Remember the Sound of Rain

1. I choose not to look at cancer as a gift but have many friends who, in this wrestling place of putting words to the incomprehensible, find comfort in viewing cancer this way. How do you view hard and difficult circumstances?

2. In what ways do you relate to Mary and/or to Martha as they stand with Jesus outside the tomb of their brother?

3. When do you struggle with words from the Evil Whisperer who raises doubts about Jesus as God, all power, and Jesus as God, all compassion? How has Jesus shown Himself to be both?

Chapter 12: The Narrow Place

1. Have you discovered Jesus in the narrow place?

2. How have you had to face your own mortality?

3. Where on your bumpy road have you experienced Jesus's comforting presence?

Chapter 13: The Final Solo

1. What stories have impacted your life?

2. What lessons are people learning from your pages? If you are experiencing the final pages, what words are being read from your life?

3. Victory songs are not about singing alone. When have you found that to be true?

Chapter 14: Sunrise, Sunset

1. When have you found yourself "hitting the wall"?
2. Sunrise. Sunset. Sometimes the only difference is the direction you are facing. Are you in the coming? Are you in the going?
3. When have you sensed the presence of God, who creates and forms face-to-face, cheek to cheek, breath to breath?

Chapter 15: The Bigger Shadow

1. Do you live under a shadow? Do you fear that since one bad thing happened, another may be right around the corner?
2. Has darkness ever become your familiar companion?
3. What do you do to stay under the shadow of almighty God (see Ps. 91:1)?

Chapter 16: Not Half of Two

1. In what ways are you tired of the hard place?
2. What have you found to be helpful when talking to your friends and family about your difficult reality?
3. When have you found it difficult to admit your needs to another person?

Chapter 17: When Anxious Thoughts Multiply

1. How have you struggled with anxiety?
2. Where are you living an asterisk life?
3. What promises from God are helpful for you to remember when you are afraid?

Chapter 18: The Dance of Surrender

1. When do you struggle to find the steps in this new dance?
2. What losses have been the most difficult to surrender?
3. Can you reach your hand to Jesus as He asks, "May I have this dance?"

Chapter 19: A Mystery Bigger than the Unanswerable

1. What are you carrying that is too difficult for you?
2. What awkward advice have people given you on your journey?
3. Do you find it comforting to picture God as a mystery bigger than the unanswerable? When have you encountered God in that way?

Chapter 20: The Most Brave

1. I write about my mom having a diagnosis of a limited number of days, but in reality, even without cancer, we all live such a life. What helps you accept this reality?
2. What are the fragile moments you are enjoying in this season?
3. For what purposes has God placed you on this earth? How are you fulfilling those purposes?

Chapter 21: Finding God in Community

1. How have you felt compelled to leave a witness of your life?
2. When have you struggled to find the smallest evidence of God's love?
3. When have you witnessed God's love in other people?

Chapter 22: The Bully in the Mirror

1. How have you faced the bully who makes daily demands for your lunch money?
2. What message do you hear when you look in the mirror?
3. By wearing lipstick, my mom refused to allow cancer to define her beauty. How have you refused to allow your hard reality to define you?

Chapter 23: When Foundations Shake

1. When have you had a day where the dominoes kept toppling, and it was too much?
2. When has someone extended timely kindness to you?
3. How has the power of kindness turned you back to God?

Chapter 24: The Gethsemane Hour

1. When have you experienced the love of others who simply chose to be there with you?
2. Have you had a Gethsemane Hour where you have pled "may this cup pass from me"?
3. Have you discovered the shade of God in the compassion of others?

Chapter 25: An Ordinary Life

1. What are your thoughts on pain and suffering? Where do you find beauty in life, despite pain and suffering? How does this point you to God?
2. What list of accomplishments would you write about your life?
3. Who handed a baton to you? To whom will you hand a baton?

Chapter 26: Chocolate Rain

1. What says "welcome home" to you?

2. How would you answer if someone asked, "Is there anything you need?"

3. Have you experienced a time when another person's love allowed you to see God's love? What was the experience?

Chapter 27: The Better Offer

1. What are your thoughts regarding the difficult realities of this life being a "momentary, light affliction"?

2. Do you find comfort in viewing death as all that is mortal being "swallowed up by life," as recorded in 2 Corinthians 5:4?

3. Can you believe and trust that Jesus will be with you when you find yourself in a hard place, even when facing death? Can you believe and trust that Jesus will also be with those you love?

Chapter 28: No More Good-Byes

1. Where have you experienced difficult good-byes?

2. Where do you find beauty in your desert journey?

3. What brings you peace in knowing God is planning a huge party in heaven?

Scriptures for Desert Sojourners

When You Are Afraid

- "Do not be afraid. . . . I have called you by name; you are mine" (Isa. 43:1 NLT).
- "Do not be anxious about anything, but in every situation, by prayer and petition, with thanksgiving, present your requests to God. And the peace of God, which transcends all understanding, will guard your hearts and minds in Christ Jesus" (Phil. 4:6–7 NIV).
- "The LORD is my light and my salvation—whom shall I fear? The LORD is the stronghold of my life—of whom shall I be afraid?" (Ps. 27:1 NIV).
- "God is our refuge and strength, an ever-present help in trouble. Therefore we will not fear, though the earth give way and the mountains fall into the heart of the sea" (Ps. 46:1–2 NIV).

When You Need Hope

- "'For I know the plans I have for you,' declares the LORD, 'plans to prosper you and not to harm you, plans to give you hope and a future'" (Jer. 29:11 NIV).

- "Rejoice in our confident hope. Be patient in trouble, and keep on praying" (Rom. 12:12 NLT).
- "This hope we have as an anchor of the soul, a hope both sure and steadfast and one which enters within the veil, where Jesus has entered as a forerunner for us" (Heb. 6:19–20).

When You Feel Alone

- "Where can I go from your Spirit? Where can I flee from your presence? If I go up to the heavens, you are there; if I make my bed in the depths, you are there" (Ps. 139:7–8 NIV).
- "Are not five sparrows sold for two pennies? Yet not one of them is forgotten by God. Indeed, the very hairs of your head are all numbered. Don't be afraid; you are worth more than many sparrows" (Luke 12:6–7 NIV).
- "And be sure of this: I am with you always, even to the end of the age" (Matt. 28:20 NLT).

When You Are in a Hard Place

- "When you go through deep waters, I will be with you. When you go through rivers of difficulty, you will not drown. . . . For I am the LORD your God" (Isa. 43:2–3 NLT).
- "At present we do not yet see all things under his control, but we see Jesus" (Heb. 2:8b–9 NET).
- "For the LORD will have compassion on Zion, have compassion on all her ruins. He will make her wilderness like Eden, and her deserts like the garden of the LORD. Joy and gladness will be found in her, thanksgiving, and the sound of singing. Sorrow and sighing will flee away" (Isa. 51:3 ISV).

When You Need to Be Reminded of the Bigness of God

- "Your eyes have seen my unformed substance; and in Your book were all written the days that were ordained for me, when as yet there was not one of them" (Ps. 139:16).
- "He counts the number of the stars; He gives names to all of them. Great is our Lord and abundant in strength; His understanding is infinite" (Ps. 147:4–5).
- "Who among all these does not know that the hand of the LORD has done this, in whose hand is the life of every living thing, and the breath of all mankind?" (Job 12:9–10).
- "'Am I a God who is near,' declares the LORD, 'and not a God far off? Can a man hide himself in hiding places so I do not see him?' declares the LORD. 'Do I not fill the heavens and the earth?' declares the LORD" (Jer. 23:23–24).

When You Need to Be Reminded of a God Who Loves

- "The LORD will command His lovingkindness in the daytime; and His song will be with me in the night, a prayer to the God of my life" (Ps. 42:8).
- "When I said, 'My foot is slipping,' your unfailing love, LORD, supported me. When anxiety was great within me, your consolation brought me joy" (Ps. 94:18–19 NIV).
- "I have loved you with an everlasting love; I have drawn you with unfailing kindness" (Jer. 31:3 NIV).
- "And so we know and rely on the love God has for us. God is love. Whoever lives in love lives in God, and God in them" (1 John 4:16 NIV).

243

When You Need to Hold On to Kindness

- "Do not let kindness and truth leave you; bind them around your neck, write them on the tablet of your heart" (Prov. 3:3).
- "Do not withhold good from those to whom it is due, when it is in your power to act" (Prov. 3:27 NIV).
- "Or do you think lightly of the riches of His kindness and tolerance and patience, not knowing that the kindness of God leads you to repentance?" (Rom. 2:4).

When You Witness Suffering

- "Weep with those who weep" (Rom. 12:15 ESV).
- "I was sick and you visited me" (Matt. 25:36 ESV).
- "For momentary, light affliction is producing for us an eternal weight of glory far beyond all comparison, while we look not at the things which are seen, but at the things which are not seen; for the things which are seen are temporal, but the things which are not seen are eternal" (2 Cor. 4:17–18).
- "For indeed while we are in this tent, we groan, being burdened, because we do not want to be unclothed but to be clothed, so that what is mortal will be swallowed up by life" (2 Cor. 5:4).

When You Need Strength

- "But they that wait upon the LORD shall renew their strength; they shall mount up with wings as eagles; they shall run, and not be weary; and they shall walk, and not faint" (Isa. 40:31 KJV).
- "The LORD is the strength of my life; of whom will I be afraid" (Ps. 27:1 ISV).
- "So do not fear, for I am with you; do not be dismayed, for I am your God. I will strengthen you and help you; I will uphold you with my righteous right hand" (Isa. 41:10 NIV).

- "My flesh and my heart may fail, but God is the strength of my heart and my portion forever" (Ps. 73:26 NIV).

When You Wrestle with Surrender

- "O LORD, my heart is not proud, nor my eyes haughty; nor do I involve myself in great matters, or in things too difficult for me. Surely I have composed and quieted my soul; like a weaned child rests against his mother, my soul is like a weaned child within me" (Ps. 131:1–2).
- "Trust in the LORD with all your heart and lean not on your own understanding; in all your ways submit to him, and he will make your paths straight" (Prov. 3:5–6 NIV).
- "He who dwells in the shelter of the Most High, will abide in the shadow of the Almighty. I will say to the LORD, 'My refuge and my fortress, my God, in whom I trust!'" (Ps. 91:1–2).

When You Face Death

- "Jesus said to her, 'I am the resurrection and the life; he who believes in Me will live even if he dies'" (John 11:25).
- "Even though I walk through the valley of the shadow of death, I fear no evil, for You are with me" (Ps. 23:4).
- "When the perishable has been clothed with the imperishable, and the mortal with immortality, then the saying that is written will come true: 'Death has been swallowed up in victory'" (1 Cor. 15:54 NIV).
- "For I am convinced that neither death nor life, neither angels nor demons, neither the present nor the future, nor any powers, neither height nor depth, nor anything else in all creation, will be able to separate us from the love of God that is in Christ Jesus our Lord" (Rom. 8:38–39 NIV).

When You Need Reminding about a Life Beyond This Life

- "At present we are men looking at puzzling reflections in a mirror. The time will come when we shall see reality whole and face to face! At present all I know is a little fraction of the truth, but the time will come when I shall know it as fully as God now knows me!" (1 Cor. 13:12 Phillips).

- "However, as it is written: 'What no eye has seen, what no ear has heard, and what no human mind has conceived—the things God has prepared for those who love him'" (1 Cor. 2:9 NIV).

- "I heard a loud shout from the throne, saying, 'Look, God's home is now among his people! He will live with them, and they will be his people. God himself will be with them. He will wipe every tear from their eyes, and there will be no more death or sorrow or crying or pain. All these things are gone forever'" (Rev. 21:3–4 NLT).

- "Praise be to the God and Father of our Lord Jesus Christ! In his great mercy he has given us new birth into a living hope through the resurrection of Jesus Christ from the dead, and into an inheritance that can never perish, spoil or fade. This inheritance is kept in heaven for you" (1 Pet. 1:3–4 NIV).

- "My Father's house has many rooms; if that were not so, would I have told you that I am going there to prepare a place for you? And if I go and prepare a place for you, I will come back and take you to be with me that you also may be where I am" (John 14:2–3 NIV).

Notes

Acknowledgments

1. Matthew 25:36 ESV.

Chapter 1 Cancer Makes a House Call

1. Numbers 21:5 NLT.
2. Exodus 13:22.
3. Mary DeMuth, *Thin Places: A Memoir* (Grand Rapids: Zondervan, 2010). Kindle edition, 11.
4. Ann Haymond Zwinger, *The Mysterious Land* (Tucson: University of Arizona Press, 1989), 5.

Chapter 2 Stupid Strong

1. Geralyn Lucas, *Why I Wore Lipstick to My Mastectomy* (New York: St. Martin's Press, 2004), 7. The author's list influenced my own.

Chapter 3 When Theology Has No Handhold

1. "Cacti" is the preferred plural spelling, according to Merriam-Webster's Dictionary, but "cactus" is acceptable and the only word I ever use.
2. Portions of this story first appeared in "How Do I Stop Being Paranoid about Cancer," www.IHadCancer.com, April 14, 2016, https://www.ihadcancer .com/h3-blog/04-14-2016/paranoid-about-cancer.
3. Betty Reid, Megan Boehnke, and Lily Leung, "Hundreds Evacuated Near Grand Canyon after Flooding," *The Arizona Republic*, August 17, 2008, http:// www.azcentral.com/news/articles/2008/08/17/20080817supai0817online.html.
4. Arthur W. Frank, *The Wounded Storyteller* (Chicago: University of Chicago Press, 2013), 80.

Chapter 4 I Will Live until I Die

1. C. S. Lewis, *Mere Christianity* (New York: HarperOne, 1980), 136.

Chapter 5 Allee, Allee, All Come Free

1. Genesis 3:9.
2. Frank, *Wounded Storyteller*, 30.

Chapter 6 Love in the Bending Low

1. "Tonto Natural Bridge State Park," Arizona State Parks, 2012, accessed July 12, 2014, http://azstateparks.com/Parks/TONA.

Chapter 7 A Hard, Forgetting Place

1. Dictionary.com, s.v. "haboob," accessed October 5, 2016, http://dictionary.reference.com/browse/haboob.
2. "Phoenix Dust Storm: Arizona Hit with Monstrous 'Haboob,'" *Huffington Post,* July 6, 2011, http://www.huffingtonpost.com/2011/07/06/phoenix-dust-storm-photos-video_n_891157.html.
3. See Matthew 14:22–33.
4. Macrina Wiederkehr, *Abide: Keeping Vigil with the Word of God* (Collegeville, MN: Liturgical Press, 2011), 91. The author's list of meanwhiles inspired me to create a list of my own.
5. Ibid., 92.
6. Jennifer Kennedy Dean, *The Power of Small: Think Small to Live Large* (Birmingham, AL: New Hope Publishers, 2011), 26.

Chapter 8 Difficult Beauty

1. Macrina Wiederkehr, *Seven Sacred Pauses: Living Mindfully through the Hours of the Day* (Notre Dame, IN: Sorin Books, 2008), 77.
2. Craig Childs, *The Secret Knowledge of Water* (New York: Little, Brown and Company, 2000), xii.
3. Hosea 2:14 NLT.
4. Craig Childs, *The Southwest's Contrary Land: Forever Changing between Four Corners and the Sea of Cortes* (Phoenix: Arizona Highways Books, 2001), 147.
5. See Matthew 4:1–11.

Chapter 9 A Stack of Gratitude Stones

1. Hebrews 2:8 NET.
2. Hebrews 2:9 NIV.
3. Ann Voskamp, "Why the Best Response to Life, The Holidays, Anything Is: Yada, Yada, Yada," *A Holy Experience*, November 11, 2013, http://www.aholyexperience.com/2013/11/why-the-best-response-to-life-the-holidays-anything-is-yada-yada-yada/.

Chapter 10 Laughter and Faith Hold Hands

1. Proverbs 17:22.

Chapter 11 Remember the Sound of Rain

1. Ken Gire, *Moments with the Savior: A Devotional Life of Christ* (Grand Rapids: Zondervan, 1998), 250–51.

2. Ibid.

3. Oswald Chambers, *My Utmost for His Highest* (Westwood, New Jersey: Barbour and Company, 1963), 211.

4. Ann Voskamp, *The Greatest Gift* (Carol Stream, IL: Tyndale House, 2013), 201.

5. Elie Wiesel from an interview with *The Bostonia*, quoted by Michael Reagan, *Inside the Mind of God: Images and Words of Inner Space* (West Conshohocken, PA: Templeton Press, 2002), 129.

6. Jennifer Kennedy Dean, *Pursuing the Christ: 31 Morning and Evening Prayers for Christmastime* (Birmingham: New Hope Publishers, 2008), 55.

Chapter 12 The Narrow Place

1. Adapted from a story my dad, Stan Hankins, wrote and gave to his mother for a Christmas present the following year, in 1978.

2. Isaiah 40:31 KJV.

3. See Isaiah 54:4–5.

Chapter 13 The Final Solo

1. Philip Yancey, *Prayer: Does It Make Any Difference?* (Grand Rapids: Zondervan, 2006), Kindle edition.

2. Luke 15:11.

3. Luke 18:10.

4. Luke 10:30.

5. Adam S. McHugh, *The Listening Life* (Downers Grove, IL: InterVarsity, 2015), 81.

6. Mark Labberton, *The Dangerous Act of Loving Your Neighbor: Seeing Others through the Eyes of Jesus* (Downers Grove, IL: InterVarsity, 2010), 163.

7. After being diagnosed with pancreatic cancer, Professor Randy Pausch gave a final lecture, which became an internet sensation and the bestselling book *The Last Lecture*.

8. Charles Hutchinson Gabriel and Civilla Durfee Martin, *His Eye Is on the Sparrow*, 1905, public domain.

9. Ibid.

Chapter 14 Sunrise, Sunset

1. Kathleen Jo Ryan, *Writing Down the River: Into the Heart of the Grand Canyon* (Flagstaff, AZ: Northland Publishing, 1998), xvii.

2. Ruth Kirk, "Of Walls and Time," in Ryan, *Writing Down the River*, 60.

3. Craig Childs, *Grand Canyon: Time below the Rim* (Phoenix: Arizona Highways Books, 1999), 129.
4. Wiederkehr, *Abide*, 24.
5. Ibid, 49.

Chapter 15 The Bigger Shadow

1. Carolina A. Miranda et al., *Discover Peru: Experience the Best of Peru* (Oakland, CA: Lonely Planet, 2011), 113.
2. "News and Updates for El Misti Volcano," August 29, 2012, https://www.volcanodiscovery.com/el-misti/news.html.
3. Ibid.
4. Lynn Eib, *Finding the Light in Cancer's Shadow* (Carol Stream, IL: Tyndale, 2006), xiv.
5. Ibid.
6. *Wikipedia*, s.v. "sillar," accessed October 11, 2016, http://en.wikipedia.org/wiki/Sillar.

Chapter 16 Not Half of Two

1. Portions of this story first appeared in Lynne Hartke, "The Rattlesnake Man," *The Gila River Review* (Fall 2010), http://www.cgc.maricopa.edu/academics/english/GilaRiverReview/Fall2010/Pages/harke2.aspx.
2. "Gila Monster," Smithsonian National Zoo and Conservation Biology Institute, accessed October 28, 2016, https://nationalzoo.si.edu/animals/gila-monster.
3. Jordan Sonnenblick, *Drums, Girls, and Dangerous Pie* (New York: Scholastic Inc. 2004).

Chapter 17 When Anxious Thoughts Multiply

1. Dictionary.com, s.v. "anxious," accessed June 27, 2014, http://dictionary.reference.com/browse/anxious.
2. Dictionary.com, s.v. "consolation," accessed June 27, 2014, http://dictionary.reference.com/browse/consolation.
3. Dutch Sheets and Chris Jackson, *Praying through Sorrows* (Shippensburg, PA: Destiny Image Publishers, 2005), 64.

Chapter 18 The Dance of Surrender

1. Sarah Young, *Jesus Calling* (Nashville: Thomas Nelson, 2011), 170.
2. Frank, *Wounded Storyteller*, 55.
3. Judson W. Van DeVenter and Winfield S. Weeden, "I Surrender All," 1896, public domain.

Chapter 19 A Mystery Bigger than the Unanswerable

1. C. S. Lewis, *A Grief Observed*, in *The Complete C. S. Lewis Signature Classics* (New York: HarperCollins, 2002), 658.

2. Sheets and Jackson, *Praying through Sorrows*, 11.

3. John Wessells, *Conversations with the Voiceless* (Grand Rapids: Zondervan, 2004), 21.

Chapter 20 The Most Brave

1. Brenda Z. Guiberson, *Cactus Hotel* (New York: Henry Holt and Company, 1991). A fantastic children's book about saguaros. Illustrated by Megan Lloyd.

2. Roy Lessin, quoted by Richard Swenson, *A Minute of Margin: Restoring Balance to Busy Lives* (Colorado Springs: NavPress, 2003), 19.

3. Frederick Turner, *Of Chiles, Cacti, and Fighting Cocks: Notes on the American West* (Markham, Ontario: North Point Press, 1990), 86.

Chapter 21 Finding God in Community

1. *Shall We Dance?* DVD. Directed by Peter Chelsom. Santa Monica, CA: Miramax Lionsgate, 2004.

2. Swenson, *A Minute of Margin*, 60.

3. Paul Brand and Philip Yancey, *In the Likeness of God* (Grand Rapids: Zondervan, 2004), 143.

4. Ibid.

5. Ibid., 138.

6. Kay Warren, *Dangerous Surrender* (Grand Rapids: Zondervan, 2007), 138.

7. C. S. Lewis, "The Problem of Pain," in *The Complete C. S. Lewis Signature Classics* (New York: HarperCollins Publisher, 2002), 613.

8. Sheets and Jackson, *Praying through Sorrows*, 152.

Chapter 22 The Bully in the Mirror

1. Edward Abbey, *The Journey Home*, (New York: Penguin Books, 1977), 14.

2. See 2 Corinthians 12:7–8.

3. Rob Bell, *Sex God: Exploring the Endless Connections between Sexuality and Spirituality* (Grand Rapids: Zondervan, 2007), 30. Bell writes, "I first came across Gonin's diary in the manifesto of the legendary British graffiti artist named Banksy, whom you must get to know (Banksy.co.uk). He cites the Imperial War Museum as his source for the diary (Bansky, Wall and Piece)."

4. Ibid.

Chapter 23 When Foundations Shake

1. Marty Gibson, *Ahwatukee Foothills News*, December 2008, quoted in Sredfield, "Lost Camp Loop," January 20, 2010, http://hikearizona.com/decoder.php?ZTN=3049. In an email dated July 21, 2016, Martin Gibson confirmed the quote was from his column published in the newspaper in December 2008, but could not confirm the exact date. The Chandler Library and newspaper no longer have digital copies for those years.

2. Hiram Bingham, "In the Wonderland of Peru," *National Geographic,* April 1913, http://ngm.nationalgeographic.com/1913/04/machu-picchu/bingham-text.

3. John Bredar, "A Marvel of Inca Engineering," NOVA, September 1, 2009, http://www.pbs.org/wgbh/nova/ancient/wright-inca-engineering.html.

4. Mark Adams, "Machu Picchu Secrets," *National Geographic,* accessed November 11, 2015, http://travel.nationalgeographic.com/top-10/peru/machu-picchu/secrets/.

5. Bredar, "A Marvel of Inca Engineering."

6. Jeff L Brown, "Water Supply and Drainage at Machu Picchu," WaterHistory.org, accessed October 13, 2016, http://www.waterhistory.org/histories/machu/.

7. Beth Moore, *Whispers of Hope: 10 Weeks of Devotional Prayer* (Nashville: Broadman & Holman, 2011), 169.

8. Ibid.

Chapter 24 The Gethsemane Hour

1. See Matthew 26:39.

2. Psalm 91:1 KJV.

Chapter 25 An Ordinary Life

1. "Doctor Who: Vincent and the Doctor," IMDb, October 14, 2016, http://www.imdb.com/title/tt1591786/quotes.

2. Elisabeth Elliot, *A Path through Suffering: Discovering the Relationship between God's Mercy and Our Pain* (Ann Arbor, MI: Servant Publications, 1990), 53.

3. Ibid.

4. Lewis, "The Problem of Pain," 613.

5. Chambers, *Utmost for His Highest,* 255.

Chapter 28 No More Good-Byes

1. Sheets and Jackson, *Praying through Sorrows,* 30. This entire section was influenced by the authors' thoughts on the significance of Mary and the first questions asked after Jesus's resurrection.

2. Max Lucado, *You'll Get through This* (Nashville: Thomas Nelson, 2013), 132.

3. Ibid. I have often said that our hearts are not created to say good-bye and found my words echoed by Max Lucado. His thoughts influenced this section.

4. Kurt Nassau, *Experimenting with Color* (New York: Franklin Watts, 1997), 54.

5. See 1 Corinthians 13:12.

Lynne Hartke celebrates the difficult and the beautiful with her husband, Kevin, in Chandler, Arizona, where they have pastored a church for more than thirty years. When not on the trails avoiding rattlesnakes, Lynne is blogging, volunteering for the American Cancer Society and Relay for Life, and keeping up with their four grown children and three grandchildren. Her upcoming calendar includes plans to hike Yosemite's Half Dome, Angels Landing in Zion National Park, and the Trans-Catalina Trail—because cancer taught her to grab on to life with both hands.

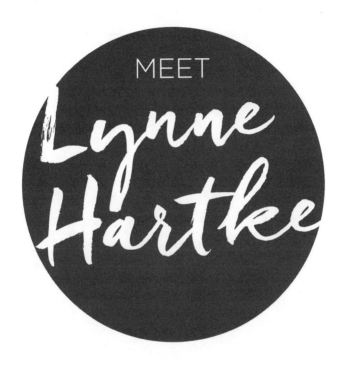

MEET

Lynne Hartke

LynneHartke.com

𝕏 @LynneHartke
f Lynne Hartke, Author